Remember your loved ones, share memories, write them down. Pass them on.
Books With Soul® is a trademark brand and supports all Authors and copywrite.
Check out our full line of books amazon.com/author/bookswithsoul
Isbn: 978-1-949325-57-7

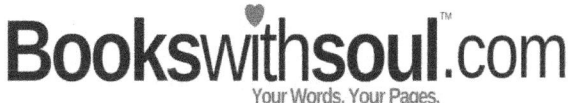

"Wherever a beautiful soul has been there is a trail of beautiful memories"

-- Author Unknown

A memory book "Remember when?"

Please pick a page and write a memory

You taught me this...

I will never forget...

You and I went here... together and I remember...

Remember When...

5 things I love about you...

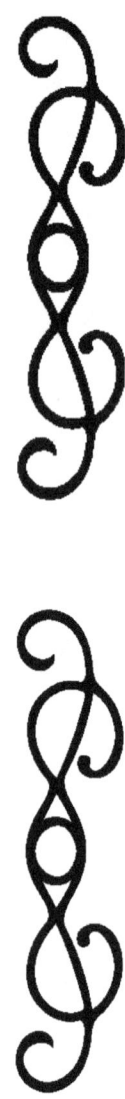

You make me laugh, especially when I think of this...

I remember you told me...

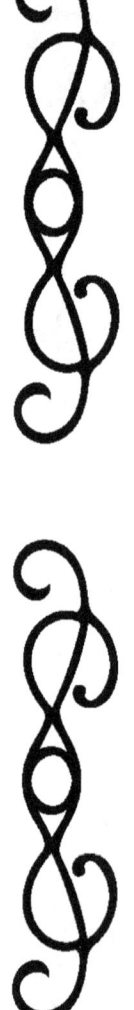

Remember the time...

Oh this was funny...

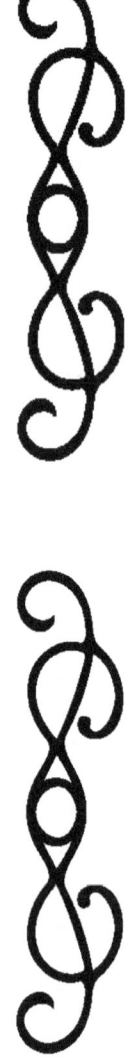

"To live in hearts we leave behind is not to die."

— Thomas Campbell

I will never forget...

You and I went here... together and I remember...

Remember When...

5 things I love about you...

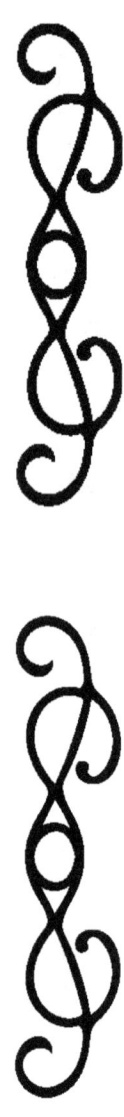

You make me laugh, especially when I think of this...

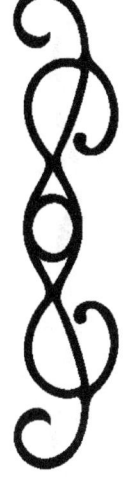

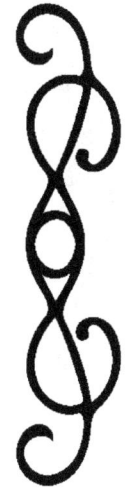

You make me laugh, especially when I think of this...

I remember you told me...

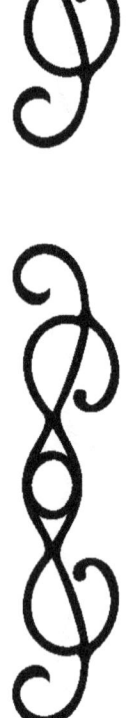

Remember the time...

Oh this was funny...

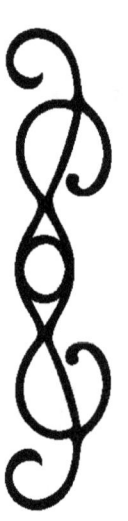

Remember the time...

5 things I love about you...

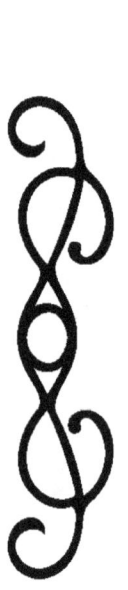

"When you lose someone you love,
you gain an angel you know"

-- Author Unknown

I will never forget...

You and I went here... together and I remember...

Remember When...

5 things I love about you...

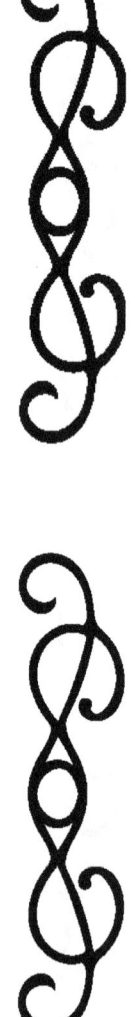

You make me laugh, especially when I think of this...

I remember you told me...

Remember the time...

Oh this was funny...

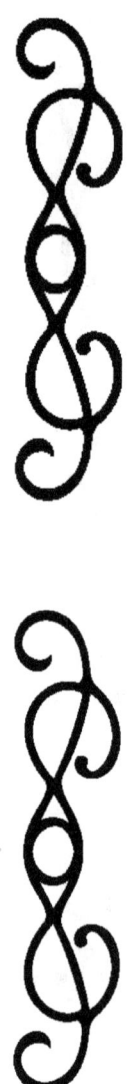

Remember the time...

5 things I love about you...

"Some people come into our lives,
leave footprints on our hearts,
and we are never the same."

-- Author Unknown

I will never forget...

You and I went here... together and I remember...

Remember When...

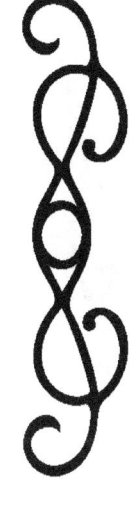
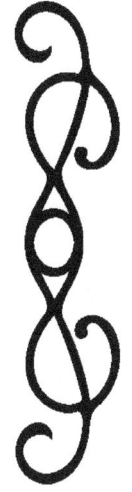

5 things I love about you...

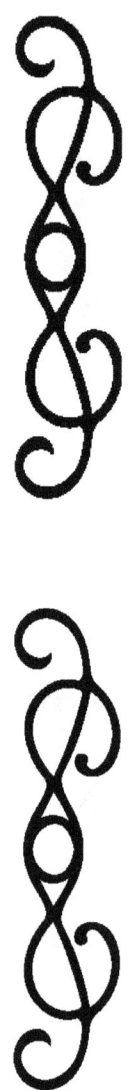

You make me laugh, especially when I think of this...

I remember you told me...

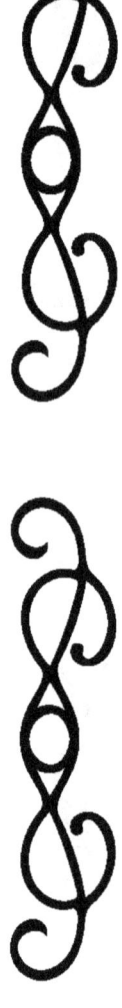

Remember the time...

Oh this was funny...

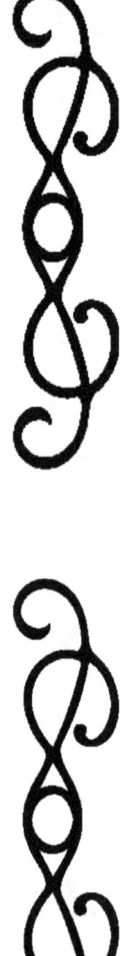

Remember the time...

5 things I love about you...

"Death leaves a heartache no one can heal,
Love leaves a memory no one can steal."

-- From a headstone in Ireland

I will never forget...

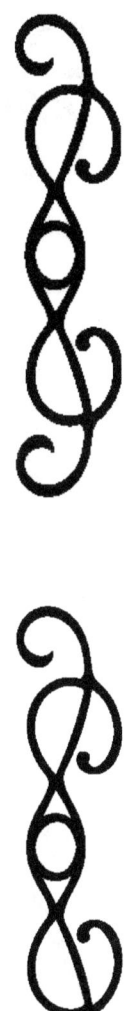

You and I went here... together and I remember...

Remember When...

5 things I love about you...

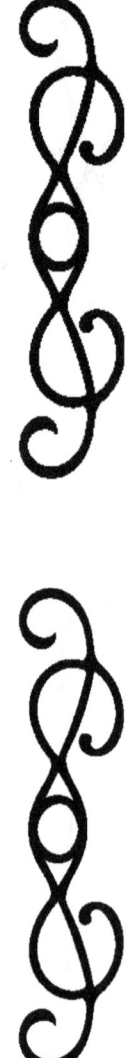

You make me laugh, especially when I think of this...

I remember you told me...

Remember the time...

Oh this was funny...

Remember the time...

5 things I love about you...

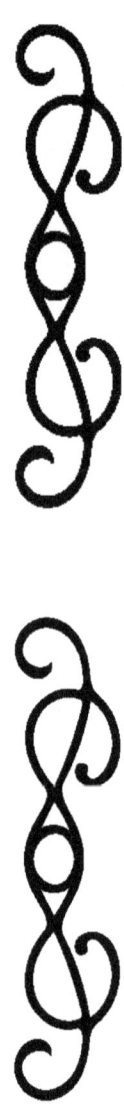

"It is not length of life, but depth of life."

-- And what a great life

I will never forget...

You and I went here... together and I remember...

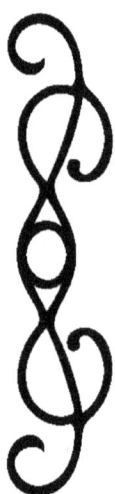

You and I went here... together and I remember...

Remember When...

5 things I love about you...

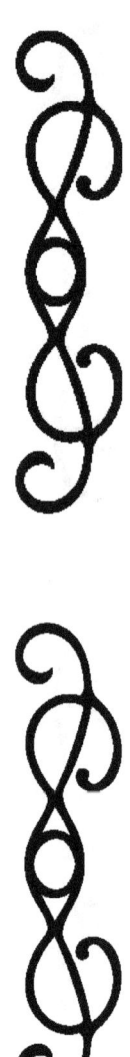

You make me laugh, especially when I think of this...

I remember you told me...

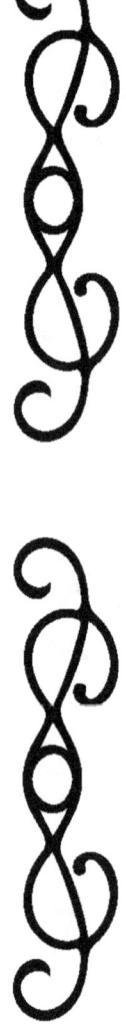

Remember the time...

Oh this was funny...

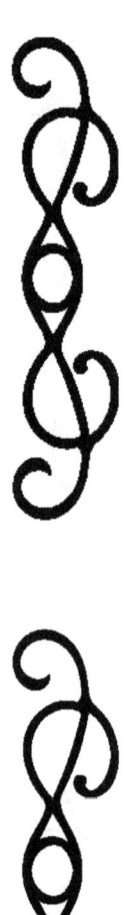

Remember the time...

5 things I love about you...

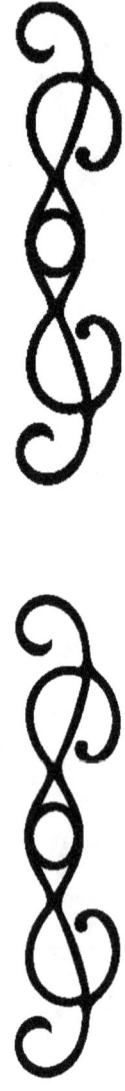

Those we have held in our arms, we hold in our hearts forever

— Author Unknown

I will never forget...

You and I went here... together and I remember...

Remember When...

5 things I love about you...

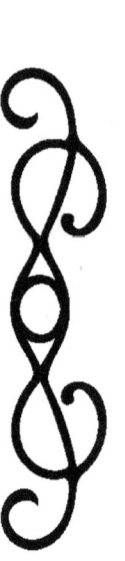

You make me laugh, especially when I think of this...

I remember you told me...

Remember the time...

Oh this was funny...

Remember the time...

5 things I love about you...

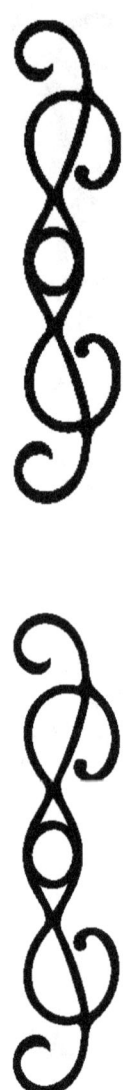

"Perhaps they are not stars in the sky,
but rather openings where our loved ones shine down
to let us know they are happy."

-- Author Unknown

I will never forget...

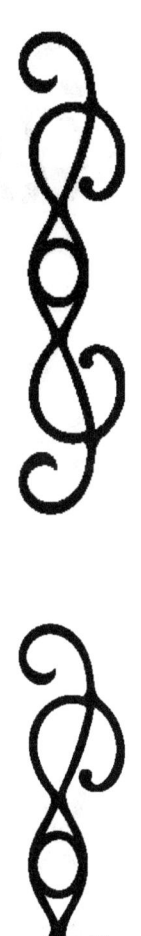

You and I went here... together and I remember...

Remember When...

5 things I love about you...

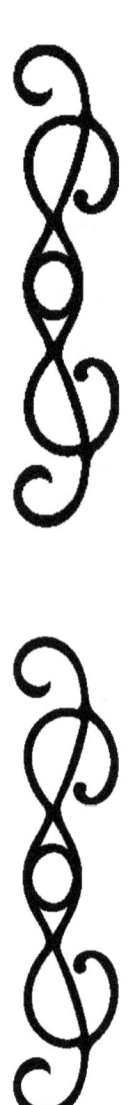

You make me laugh, especially when I think of this...

I remember you told me...

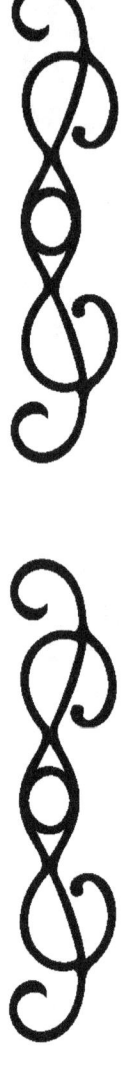

Remember the time...

Oh this was funny...

Remember the time...

5 things I love about you...

Like a bird singing in the rain,
let grateful memories survive in time
of sorrow.

-- Robert Louis Stevenson

I will never forget...

You and I went here... together and I remember...

Remember When...

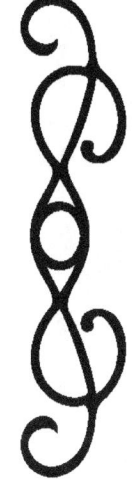
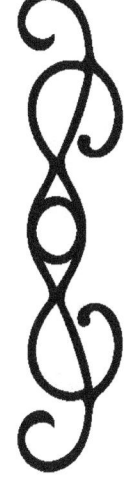

5 things I love about you...

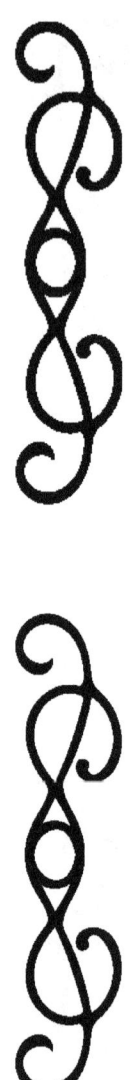

You make me laugh, especially when I think of this...

I remember you told me...

Remember the time...

Oh this was funny...

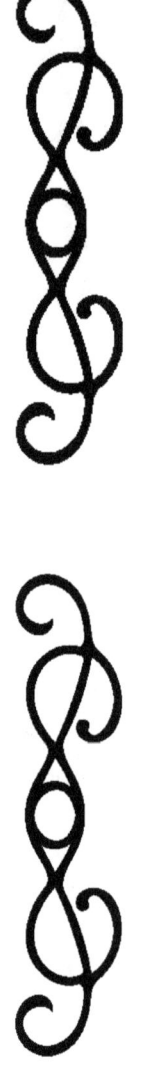

Remember the time...

5 things I love about you...

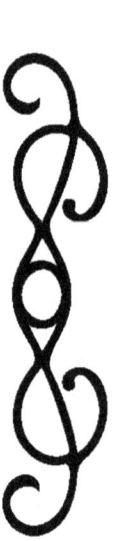

"For death is no more than a turning of us over from time to eternity."

-- William Penn

I will never forget...

You and I went here... together and I remember...

Remember When...

5 things I love about you...

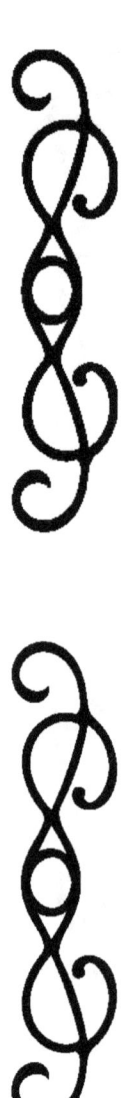

You make me laugh, especially when I think of this...

I remember you told me...

Remember the time...

Oh this was funny...

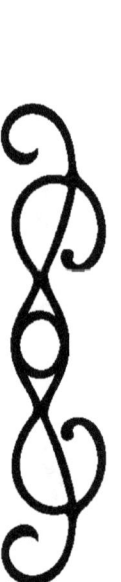

Remember the time...

5 things I love about you...

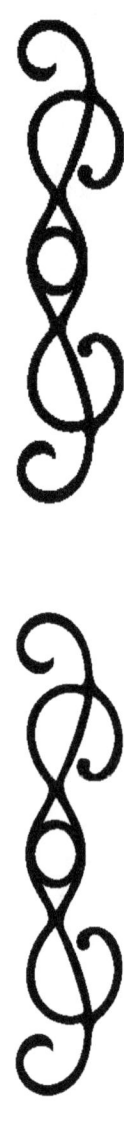

"In the end, it's not the years in your life that count. It's the life in your years.

-- Abraham Lincoln

CPSIA information can be obtained
at www.ICGtesting.com
Printed in the USA
BVHW011201190321
602998BV00007B/142

The Plant-Based Fitness Cookbook for Women Above 60 [3 in 1]

Eat Dozens of Delicious Plant-Based Dishes, Customize Your Workouts and Regain Your Lost Shape!

Anphora Cooper

Text Copyright © Anphora Cooper

All rights reserved. No part of this guide may be reproduced in any form without permission in writing from the publisher except in the case of brief quotations embodied in critical articles or reviews.

Legal & Disclaimer

The information contained in this book and its contents is not designed to replace or take the place of any form of medical or professional advice; and is not meant to replace the need for independent medical, financial, legal or other professional advice or services, as may be required. The content and information in this book has been provided for educational and entertainment purposes only.

The content and information contained in this book has been compiled from sources deemed reliable, and it is accurate to the best of the Author's knowledge, information and belief. However, the Author cannot guarantee its accuracy and validity and cannot be held liable for any errors and/or omissions. Further, changes are periodically made to this book as and when needed. Where appropriate and/or necessary, you must consult a professional (including but not limited to your doctor, attorney, financial advisor or such other professional advisor) before using any of the suggested remedies, techniques, or information in this book.

Upon using the contents and information contained in this book, you agree to hold harmless the Author from and against any damages, costs, and expenses, including any legal fees potentially resulting from the application of any of the information provided by this book. This disclaimer applies to any loss, damages or injury caused by the use and application, whether directly or indirectly, of any advice or information presented, whether for breach of contract, tort, negligence, personal injury, criminal intent, or under any other cause of action.

You agree to accept all risks of using the information presented inside this book.

You agree that by continuing to read this book, where appropriate and/or necessary, you shall consult a professional (including but not limited to your doctor, attorney, or financial advisor or such other advisor as needed) before using any of the suggested remedies, techniques, or information in this book.

Contents

The Plant-Based Diet Cookbook with Pictures

Introduction:	17
WHAT IS A WHOLE-FOOD, PLANT-BASED DIET?	19
What Makes Plant-based Diets So Healthy?	20
THE FIVE FOOD GROUPS	21
THE BENEFITS OF A WHOLE-FOOD, PLANT-BASED DIET	26
Plant-Based Diet Kick Start Guide	28
Recipes for plant-based dishes	31
Breakfast:	31
1. Protein boost loaf	31
2. Mixed-up Seed Bread DRY	34
3. Flat Bread for Tree Huggers	36
4. Quinoa Yogi-Power Porridge (serves 4)	37
5. Chia Seed Pudding (Serves 4-6)	39
6. Pancake Domination	41
7. Nutty Milks	43
8. **SMOOTHIES**	44
9. TOFU SCRAMBLE	45
10. **"FRIED" POTATOES:**	46
11. TROPICAL FRUIT SALAD WITH MINT SAUCE	47
12. Lebanese Roast Ratatouille with Hummus	48
13. **Coconut Berry Swirl**	49

14. BANANA BREAD — 50

Lunch — 52

15. A "WHAT" SALAD SANDWICH — 52
16. **GRILLED PORTOBELLO MUSHROOM AND QUINOA SALAD** — 53
17. **Andalusian Tomato Salad** — 55
18. Green Salad Supremacy — 56
19. Orange & Coriander Kindness — 58
20. Cozy Winter Salad — 59
21. **Crispy Broccolini & Chickpeas with Cashew 'Ricotta'** — 62
22. Quick Chickpea Curry — 63
23. Spiced Chickpeas with Cauli Mash — 64
24. **Red Lentils with Tomato & Spinach** — 66
25. **Zen Habits Three-Bean Veggie Chili** — 67
26. **Gentle Lentils** — 69
27. **Spiced Lentils with Hummus** — 70
28. **CHILI** — 71

Soups — 73

29. Clear Vegetable Soup — 73
30. Cauliflower Soup — 74
31. Moroccan sweet potato lentil — 75
32. Mushroom Soup — 77
33. Turmeric Tomato Detox Soup — 78
34. Instant Pot Lentil Soup — 80
35. Veggie-Packed Tomato Soup — 82
36. BROCCOLI AND RED LENTIL DETOX SOUP — 84

37.	Green Detox Soup	86
38.	**Easy Garbanzo Beans Curry Soup**	**88**
39.	Keto Broccoli Soup	90
40.	Delish and Quick Thai Soup	91
41.	Italian Vegetable Soup	93
42.	Vegetarian Collard Greens Soup	95

Dinner: 97

43.	Khichdi	97
44.	**Bulgogi-Style Eggplant**	**99**
45.	Chinese Broccoli with Soy Paste	101
46.	Red Pepper, Potato, and Peanut Sabzi	102
47.	Adobo-Style Eggplant	103
48.	Galayet Banadoura	105
49.	**Cauliflower Steaks**	**107**
50.	Eggplant Lasagna	108
51.	nasi goreng	111
52.	indian shepherd's pie	113
53.	kimchi fried rice	116
54.	aloo gobi (indian-spiced potatoes & cauliflower)	118
55.	butternut lasagna with mushrooms and sage	120
56.	Rigatoni with Easy Vodka Sauce	124

Desert; 127

57.	Vegan Apple Cake	127
58.	**Vegan Chocolate Chip Cookies**	**129**
59.	**VEGAN ALMOND JOY BAR**	**131**
60.	No-Bake Vanilla Cake Bites	132

61. Chilled Chocolate Torte	134
62. Peanut Butter Protein Balls	137
63. Cinnamon Walnut Apple Cake Baked with Olive Oil	138
64. GREEK YOGURT CHOCOLATE MOUSSE	140
65. Fig and pistachio cake	141
66. Sticky Gluten-Free Lemon Cake	143
67. Balsamic Berries with Honey Yogurt	147
68. Blood Orange Olive Oil Cake	148
69. Honeyed Phyllo Stacks with Pistachios, Spiced Fruit & Yogurt	150
70. Aztec Chocolate Granola Bark	153

The 15-Day Women's Health Book of 15-Minute Workouts

Introduction	**158**
Chapter 1: What is the 15-Minute workouts?	**160**
WORK SMARTER, NOT HARDER	160
A HEALTHIER LIFESTYLE	161
ALL YOU NEED IS YOU	162
Chapter 2: The Science of Leanness	**164**
LEANNESS IS NOT A FOUR-LETTER WORD	165
DIET	166
DIETING TIPS	167

Chapter 3: How to Maximize Post-Workout Recovery so You Can Train Harder and Recover Faster.   **171**

  MAXIMIZING POST-WORKOUT RECOVERY   174

Chapter 4: The Science of Muscular Strength   **176**

  MUSCULAR STRENGTH AND DEVELOPMENT FACTS   176

  HOW THE BODY CREATES MUSCLE   178

Chapter 5: How to Build Lean Muscle (and Raise Your Metabolism)   **180**

  SAMPLE WORKOUT SCHEDULE   183

    DAY 1: CHEST/TRICEPS (REST DAY)   184

    DAY 2: BACK/BICEPS (REST DAY)   185

    DAY 3: LEGS/CORE(REST DAY)   186

    DAY 4: CHEST/TRICEPS (REST DAY)   187

    DAY 5: BACK/BICEPS (REST DAY)   188

Chapter 6: Resize Your Thighs   **191**

  LEG AND THIGH WORKOUT 1   191

    PART A   191

    PART B   193

  LEG AND THIGH WORKOUT 2   195

  LOWER BODY WORKOUT 3   197

  LEG AND THIGH WORKOUT 4   198

    PART A   198

    PART B   198

  LEG AND THIGH WORKOUT 5   199

Chapter 7: The Lean 15-Minute Workouts for Building Muscle and Losing Fat   **200**

Chapter 8: The 15-Day Body of Your Dreams in Just 15 Minutes a Day (or Less) — 206

PART I. INTRODUCTION TO THE 15 DAY LEAN BODY PROGRAM — 206

PART II. THE FAST TRACK TO THE CORE PROGRAM — 209

PART III. THE FAST TRACK TO THE FAT BURN PROGRAM — 211

PART IV. WRAPPING UP WITH FAT-BURNING TIPS FROM OUR ALL-STAR TEAM — 213

Chapter 9: Benefits Of 15 Minutes Workout — 216

THERE ARE VARIOUS TIPS WHICH NEEDS TO BE FOLLOWED BEFORE EXERCISING — 216

Conclusion — 222

7-Minute Workout for Seniors

Introduction — 227

Chapter 1: The Benefits of Doing the 7-Minute Workout — 229

The 7-minute workout is beneficial in many ways. — 229

Benefits of doing the 7 minute workout to the old: — 230

The 7-Minute Workout for Seniors has many benefits: — 231

The three strength training exercises are: — 233

Chapter 2: How to do the 7-minute Workout — 236

Chapter 3: Three Powerful Techniques to Make Exercise a Habit — 242

Technique 1: Habit Stacking — 245

What it is: 245

How will this help me? 245

Technique 2: Conditioned Cues 245

Technique 3: Intrinsic Reward Statements 246

What is it: 247

How will it help me: 247

Key takeaways 248

Chapter 4: Great Results at Home with Little or No Equipment 249

Functional Training 249

Exercising at Home 250

Combination Approach 251

Chapter 5: The 7 Minute Workout for Seniors: Rest and Recovery 256

Early Recovery phase 256

The Late Recovery phase 257

Active Recovery, 258

Chapter 6: Tips for Family Members and Caregivers 261

Enthusiasm 262

Empathy 262

Encourage 263

Ease 264

Key Takeaways 267

Action Steps — 267

Chapter 7: The Workout Routine — 269

Here's a sample stretching, strengthening, and cardio routine. — 270

Chapter 8: Is There an Ideal Diet? — 276

Popular Diets — 277

The components of the Mediterranean diet: — 279

Food Sources: Good and Bad — 280

Chapter 9: Motivation and Commitment — 284

The Motivation — 284

The Commitment — 285

Positive Reinforcements — 286

Inspirational Quotes — 288

Chapter 10: Questions and Answers — 291

How to Improve Your Performance: — 292

Questions and answers on the 7-minute workout for the seniors: — 293

Conclusion — 299

The Plant-Based Diet Cookbook with Pictures

Tens of Vegetarian Recipes to Shed Weight and Stay Healthy in a Post-Pandemic Scenario

Anphora Cooper

Contents

Introduction: 17
WHAT IS A WHOLE-FOOD, PLANT-BASED DIET? 19
What Makes Plant-based Diets So Healthy? 20
THE FIVE FOOD GROUPS 21
THE BENEFITS OF A WHOLE-FOOD, PLANT-BASED DIET ... 26
Plant-Based Diet Kick Start Guide 28
Recipes for plant-based dishes 31

  Breakfast: 31
    1. Protein boost loaf 31
    2. Mixed-up Seed Bread DRY 34
    3. Flat Bread for Tree Huggers 36
    4. Quinoa Yogi-Power Porridge (serves 4) 37
    5. Chia Seed Pudding (Serves 4-6) 39
    6. Pancake Domination 41
    7. Nutty Milks 43
    8. **SMOOTHIES** 44
    9. TOFU SCRAMBLE 45
    10. "FRIED" POTATOES: 46
    11. TROPICAL FRUIT SALAD WITH MINT SAUCE 47
    12. Lebanese Roast Ratatouille with Hummus 48
    13. Coconut Berry Swirl 49
    14. BANANA BREAD 50

  Lunch 52

15. A "WHAT" SALAD SANDWICH 52
16. **GRILLED PORTOBELLO MUSHROOM AND QUINOA SALAD** 53
17. **Andalusian Tomato Salad** 55
18. Green Salad Supremacy 56
19. Orange & Coriander Kindness 58
20. Cozy Winter Salad 59
21. **Crispy Broccolini & Chickpeas with Cashew 'Ricotta'** 62
22. Quick Chickpea Curry 63
23. Spiced Chickpeas with Cauli Mash 64
24. **Red Lentils with Tomato & Spinach** 66
25. **Zen Habits Three-Bean Veggie Chili** 67
26. **Gentle Lentils** 69
27. **Spiced Lentils with Hummus** 70
28. **CHILI** 71

Soups 73

29. Clear Vegetable Soup 73
30. Cauliflower Soup 74
31. Moroccan sweet potato lentil 75
32. Mushroom Soup 77
33. Turmeric Tomato Detox Soup 78
34. Instant Pot Lentil Soup 80
35. Veggie-Packed Tomato Soup 82
36. BROCCOLI AND RED LENTIL DETOX SOUP 84
37. Green Detox Soup 86
38. **Easy Garbanzo Beans Curry Soup** 88

- 39. Keto Broccoli Soup 90
- 40. Delish and Quick Thai Soup 91
- 41. Italian Vegetable Soup 93
- 42. Vegetarian Collard Greens Soup 95

Dinner: 97
- 43. Khichdi 97
- **44. Bulgogi-Style Eggplant** 99
- 45. Chinese Broccoli with Soy Paste 101
- 46. Red Pepper, Potato, and Peanut Sabzi 102
- 47. Adobo-Style Eggplant 103
- 48. Galayet Banadoura 105
- **49. Cauliflower Steaks** 107
- 50. Eggplant Lasagna 108
- 51. nasi goreng 111
- 52. indian shepherd's pie 113
- 53. kimchi fried rice 116
- 54. aloo gobi (indian-spiced potatoes & cauliflower) 118
- 55. butternut lasagna with mushrooms and sage 120
- 56. Rigatoni with Easy Vodka Sauce 124

Desert; 127
- 57. Vegan Apple Cake 127
- **58. Vegan Chocolate Chip Cookies** 129
- **59. VEGAN ALMOND JOY BAR** 131
- **60. No-Bake Vanilla Cake Bites** 132
- **61. Chilled Chocolate Torte** 134
- **62. Peanut Butter Protein Balls** 137

63. **Cinnamon Walnut Apple Cake Baked with Olive Oil** .. 138
64. **GREEK YOGURT CHOCOLATE MOUSSE** 140
65. **Fig and pistachio cake** 141
66. Sticky Gluten-Free Lemon Cake 143
67. Balsamic Berries with Honey Yogurt 147
68. Blood Orange Olive Oil Cake 148
69. Honeyed Phyllo Stacks with Pistachios, Spiced Fruit & Yogurt 150
70. **Aztec Chocolate Granola Bark** 153

Introduction:

Junks and unhealthy foods are significant for different health conditions, diseases, and obesity. Numerous animal-based foods and junk meals are profoundly processed and loaded up with unneeded calories, saturated fats, added sugars, and additives that are destructive to your body and general prosperity. What we eat or don't eat influences our health and body emphatically or adversely. Somehow, diabetes, hypertension, heart diseases, liver diseases, kidney diseases, cancer, and different diseases are identified with what we eat. A whole food plant-based diet is a solid diet that centers around whole, unprocessed, or minimally processed plant foods, like tubers, legumes, whole grains, vegetables, and other plant foods, which lessens your risks of having cancer and various diseases and supports weight reduction. The plant-based diet cuts back on animal-based foods, a significant source of saturated fat and cholesterol in the omnivore's diet. A plant-based diet is an incredible choice for you on the off chance that you are worried about the danger of having cancer, on the off chance that you need to forestall Long-term diseases such as diabetes, type 2, ,and heart disease, if you need to help the planet. You morally or ethically object to eating creatures or creature items and on the off chance that you need to eliminate the carbon impression of your diet. Focusing on whole, unprocessed plant-based nourishments will help you invert and improve numerous wellbeing inconveniences, any autoimmune conditions, and excess weight. The plant-based diet is a flavorful diet with a few new rarities and plant-based transformations of your already-like nourishments. When you begin on the plant-based diet, your energy level expands, you start to lose weight, and it gets simpler as your body becomes accustomed to plant-based food sources.

WHAT IS A WHOLE-FOOD, PLANT-BASED DIET?

A whole-food, plant-based eating routine allows you to meet your nutritional requirements by focusing on natural, minimally processed plant foods, and it's based on the accompanying standards:

- **Whole foods** depict natural foods that are not heavily prepared. That implies whole, crude, or minimally refined ingredients.

- **Plant-based** implies food that comes from plants and does exclude animal ingredients like meat, milk, eggs, or honey.

What Makes Plant-based Diets So Healthy?

Besides being low in calories and plentiful in fiber, vitamins, and minerals, plant foods are stacked with a huge number of mixtures called phytonutrients ("Phyto" means plant in Greek) which go about as natural antioxidants, anti-inflammatories, and detoxifiers. These mixtures blend and match in innumerable combinations within plants to give these benefits. Instances of phytonutrients are the orange/red carotenoids in carrots and tomatoes, polyphenols in berries, tea, and dark chocolate, and phytoestrogens in soybeans. Large numbers of these mixtures give plants their shade, so varying the shades of your foods grown from the ground and eating an assortment of whole grains, nuts, seeds, and legumes naturally change these phytonutrients.

THE FIVE FOOD GROUPS

Here's a snappy outline of the significant food categories you'll enjoy on a plant-based diet, with examples:

- **Fruits:** Any kind of fruit, including apples, bananas, grapes, strawberries, citrus fruits, and so forth

- **Vegetables:** lots of vegetables, including peppers, corn, lettuce, spinach, kale, peas, collards, and so forth.

- **Tubers:** Root veggies like potatoes, carrots, parsnips, sweet potatoes, beets, and so forth.

- **Whole grains:** Grains, cereals, and different starches in their whole form, for example, Quinoa, Brown Rice, millet, whole wheat, oats, barley, and so forth even; popcorn is a whole grain.

- **Legumes:** Beans of any type, plus lentils, pulses, and so on.

There are lots of different foods you may also experience, including nuts, seeds, avocados, tofu, tempeh, whole-grain flours and bread, and plant-based milk. Be that as it may, we suggest eating these foods with some restraint can make a contribution to weight gain.

Special nutrients to consider

Protein

Protein is in each cell of the body. It is utilized to fabricate and fix muscles, bone, skin, and the immune system. We additionally need it to make hormones and enzymes. Proteins are comprised of amino acids.

Your body can make a portion of the amino acids, yet not every one of them. The ones your body can't make are called essential. Without much of a stretch, you can meet your protein needs every day from plant-based foods like nuts, peas, beans, seeds, whole grains, vegetables, and soy products.

A seed that acts like grain is known as Quinoa, is an incredible wellspring of protein and essential amino acids.

Adults need about 0.36 gm of protein per pound of body weight per day. Multiply your body-weight by 0.36 to find out how much protein you need. For instance, if your weight is 220 pounds: 220 x 0.36 = about 79.2 gm of protein per day.

B12

The human body needs vitamin B12 for the nerve functioning and also for making red blood cells. In the event that you don't get enough B12, you can create anemia or nerve damage. Most B12 comes from animal-based foods. B12 is found in some fortified foods and also in nutritional yeast, for example:

- Meat substitutes
- Cereals
- Hemp milk or rice

Read labels for these items to ensure B12 has been added.

Since it may not be not difficult to get enough B12 from fortified foods, it very well might be ideal for taking a supplement. As you get older, your body is less ready to absorb B12. Your doctor may propose a supplement or shot to help forestall a deficiency. Talk with your registered dietitian or doctor for more info.

Iron

Iron is a mineral present inside humans's blood that carries oxygen. Getting sufficient iron is significant for everybody, especially pregnant women, women of childbearing age, children, and infants. Iron-rich plant-based foods include whole-grain bread and cereals, dried beans and peas, dark green leafy vegetables, dried fruits, nuts, and seeds. A few foods, such as breakfast cereals, are fortified with iron. The sort of iron found in plant-based foods isn't absorbed as effectively as the iron in animal products. Be that as it may, eating iron-rich foods alongside vitamin C can help your body better utilize iron. A few foods with vitamin C are oranges, mangos, kiwis, strawberries, red peppers, tomatoes, broccoli, and bok choy. A few people may have to take a supplement.

Calcium

Calcium facilitates the building of bones and teeth. It is also important for the functioning of the heart, muscles, and nerves. Good assets of calcium are Chinese cabbage, bok choy, kale, calcium-set tofu, and broccoli. There also are many calcium-fortified meals, including cereal, soy and

almond milk.

Zinc

Zinc is necessary and important for the immune system wound recuperation and manages blood sugar manage. Good assets are whole grains, tofu, tempeh, beans, peas, lentils, nuts, seeds, and fortified breakfast cereals. Compounds in plant foods referred to as phytates hold zinc from being absorbed. This may be improved by soaking beans, grains, and seeds in water for numerous hours earlier than cooking. Consuming sprouted grains and beans and leavened grains, inclusive of bread, in preference to crackers also increases absorption. Some foods are fortified with zinc.

Vitamin D

Vitamin D is needed for strong bones. It is also wanted for muscle and nerves, and the immune system to work properly. Very few meals have Vitamin D. We get most of our vitamin D when the skin is exposed to the sun, but many humans do no longer make sufficient from sun exposure alone. Some foods, which include soy or almond milk and cereal, have added vitamin D. You may additionally need to take supplements. Talk with your doctor for more info.

Omega-3 Fatty Acids

Omega-3 fatty acids, which include docosahexaenoic acid (DHA) and eicosatetraenoic acid (EPA) discovered in fatty fish, may decrease the danger of heart disease and help the immune system and brain. Good sources of plant-based omega-3 fats consist of floor flaxseeds and flaxseed oil, walnuts, chia seeds, and organic canola oil. Plant-based omega-3s don't easily convert to EPA and DHA inside the body. For some human beings, which includes pregnant girls or humans with persistent health conditions, taking a micro-algae supplement can be beneficial. Ask your health Doctor for more info.

THE BENEFITS OF A WHOLE-FOOD, PLANT-BASED DIET

There are several predominant advantages to moving to plant-based nutrition, and all are supported through tremendous science. These advantages are the following:

- **Easy weight management:** Individuals who eat a plant-based diet will, in general, be less fatty than the individuals who don't, and the diet makes it easy to lose weight and keep it off—without checking calories.

- **Disease prevention:** Whole-food, plant-based eating can prevent, halt, or even reverse chronic diseases, including heart disease and type 2 diabetes.

- **A lighter environmental footprint:** A plant-based diet places much less stress on the environment.

Changing To A Plant-Based Diet

Desiring to change your diet is a start, but not enough. It is important to change gradually and change in phases. I have outlined four phases of change into a plant-based diet without upsetting your body.

The Meat Reduction Phase

Gradually reduce the meat, start with a day of the week and then, progressively ex- tend to other weekdays. Another way to do this is to get rid of red meat, chicken and turkey, fish, and other seafood in succession for 1-6 months. Importantly, work with what is comfortable for you. Once you have gotten rid of the meat, it becomes necessary for you to try out new plant-based foods that are nutritious and avoid giving in to the temptation of just filling your diet with less nutritious starches.

The Eggs Elimination Phase

Eggs are not necessarily free of unkindness and cruelty. Once you have successfully eliminated red meat, poultry, and seafood, you should also get rid of your diet's eggs, and it gets easier at this level.

The Milk and Other Dairy Products Elimination Phase

There are some milk alternatives on the plant-based diet, such as almond milk, soymilk, etc. This level can be challenging for a good number of people, given that cheese is eliminated. It is best to focus on several delicious meals which you are eating, not on the meals you are letting off.

Plant-Based Diet Kick Start Guide

Beginning on a plant-based diet can be energizing, and a bit is overpowering from the start. You start to consider how to stay on a diet eating just whole and plant-based foods, and you are frequently defied with the trouble of sorting out what to eat or not to eat. Maybe you likewise need to improve your wellbeing by improving your nutrition. Figuring out how to eat an all the more whole-food, plant-based diet will help you turn out to be better and live more. Similarly, as with numerous different diets, it is significant that you don't roll out revolutionary improvements on your diet without talking with your PCP, most particularly if you have any clinical issue or are getting treatment. The diet's adjustment affects the body, and a few medicines may need to be changed or observed within a short period.

Meal Guide

What To Eat

The following are plant-based categories to choose from and include in your meals:

Good and Healthy Starches

Eat well starches stacked with such a lot of nutrition, such as steel-cut oats, sweet potatoes, brown rice, squash, red potatoes, sprouted whole wheat, and so forth.

Vegetables and Fruits

Eat a collection of daily fruit basis, like blackberries, strawberries, beets, garlic, oranges, pears, bananas, mangoes, peaches, bell pepper, lemons, limes, apples, figs, raspberries, blueberries, celery, cauliflower, and numerous different fruits and vegetables.

Greens

Greens are a vital piece of a whole food plant-based diet, and it is essential to remember loads of them for your diet consistently. Dim, verdant green vegetables are nutritious and loaded up with iron, calcium, and loads of vitamins. Instances of greens that you can add to your day-by-day diet include collards, kale, spinach, broccoli, and lots more.

Healthy and Unsaturated Fats

Saturated fats are unhealthy fats that cause damage to the body and wellbeing. There are healthy fats that are useful for you, also called unsaturated. Fortunately, a couple of plant food sources have saturated fats. Plant nourishments with healthy unsaturated fats incorporate canola oil, olive oil, hemp seeds, chia seeds, flaxseeds, walnuts, raw almonds, and avocado.

Proteins

Beans are acceptable protein sources; for example, kidney beans, pinto beans, garbanzo beans, edamame (soybeans), lentils, and so forth. Seitan, tempeh, tofu, black beans are likewise extraordinary protein sources. Other extraordinary protein sources are organic soy yogurt, almond milk, and soy milk. Seeds and nuts are extraordinary wellsprings of protein, similar to hemp seed protein powder, chia seeds, ground flaxseeds, walnuts, and raw almonds brimming with nutrients.

Other Healthy Food Sources

As you get used to plant-based diets, you will discover more healthy food options that are plant-based, and you will discover how to put them all together seamlessly. Such food options may include spices, seasonings, nutritional yeast, spirulina, turmeric, cinnamon, green tea, red wine, etc.

Learning to combine these food options into meals is not as difficult as it may seem. With time, you will become fully acquainted with making delicious plant-based meals with little or no effort.

Recipes for plant-based dishes

Breakfast:

1. **Protein boost loaf**

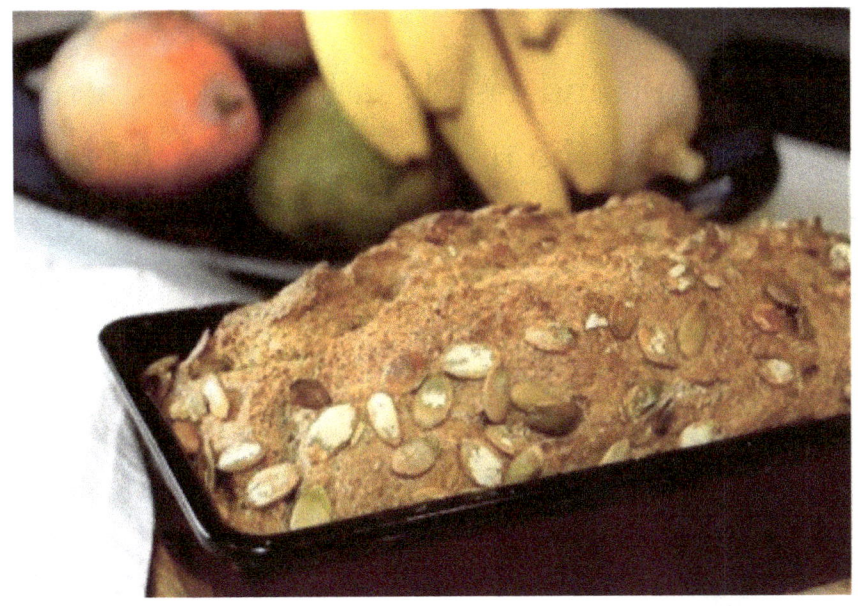

Ingredients

- 200 grams of Quinoa or Millet flour

- 100 grams of Buckwheat flour

- 100 grams whole grain Rice flour

- 1tbs Bicarbonate of Soda

- 500-700 grams of Water

- 2tbs of Salt

- 1-2 fruits like Banana, Apple or Carrot

Optional Ingredients

- 50 grams of Raisins

- 100 grams of Nuts (Almonds, Walnuts, Hazelnuts)

- 50 grams of Linseeds

This is the most forgiving and easy bread to make. Calculate 15 minutes to mix the ingredients for the dough. The thing to keep in mind is to add approximately 1tsp of bicarbonate, 1tsp of Salt, and one sweet fruit for every 5dl of flour, so make as much as you want. The sugar in the fruit and the Salt activates the bicarbonate that raises the bread. The more compact and heavier the flour you use, the more Salt, bicarbonate, and sugar (fruit) you need for the bread to raise. If you are on a diet, use carrots instead of fruit. We usually use carrots. It is so forgiving that if you bake it too fast and too hot, just lower the temperature and put it in again, maybe sliced up. If you didn't have time to bake it, keep it in the fridge and bake it later. It can even be easily frozen.

PROCESS

Mix all the ingredients in separate bowls to be sure each is well mixed. Then mix the two together until you get the consistency of a sticky porridge. You can add more water to get the right consistency if it's not sticky at first, but don't let it get runny. Flours tend to be different in different countries, so bear this in mind. If your mixture is too dry, add more water. -Place the thick porridge-like dough in bread trays. Put pumpkin, sesame, or other seeds on top if you want, and tap them down a little so they stick to the surface. -Bake for 40-60 minutes at

160C, depending on how sticky the mixture is. -Stick a probe in the center of the bread to see if it's ready. When the stick comes out clean, the bread is ready. If it comes out sticky, the bread's not ready. If you happen to take the bread out too early, just put it in again. Bread always likes to rest before being cut, so let it cool off under a towel for about 20 minutes before eating (if you can). We also like to switch off the oven and let it cook in the after heat. Tips! Freeze all the "old" bananas and other fruit you don't get around to eating because you can use them for this bread or as sweeteners in healthy desserts. When the fruit turns old, it produces more fructose (the sugar in fruit), and that's why it becomes sweeter with time. But as we have learned, don't forget to peel the fruit before freezing! If you don't have time to bake the bread after making the dough, just leave the dough in the fridge and bake it whenever you have the time. We often leave the dough overnight and bake it in the morning so that we have newly baked bread to start the day. We do all the time. It's a very "forgiving" bread, and you can elaborate a lot until you find exactly what you like, but DON'T falls into the trap of using white wheat flour. Then you miss the whole point and might as well buy a white, pre-sliced, nutrient-free loaf from the supermarket. Quick **Note on** Nuts and Soaked Nuts A nut wants to fall into wet soil to grow the plant it was meant to produce. When the nut comes into contact with water, the hard outer shell opens, the nut gets wet, and it "comes alive" from its dormant phase. Nature has protected nuts from animals or bugs with a bitter taste and peal, which is usually enough for predators to leave them lying on the ground. It's also what makes some people have trouble digesting them. These bitter enzymes are dissolved when the nuts are soaked in water. They also develop dormant enzymes to strengthen the little plant-to-be. This means that minerals and other good nutrients are bioavailable, and the nut also becomes much healthier and easier to digest for us humans. When we toast nuts, the bitter enzymes and taste go away, but it also kills the enzymes that make them so nutritious. Still, however, lightly toasted nuts could still be healthy for us, though deep-fried and salted nuts are not. The best is to soak nuts. Just leave them for a few hours or over-night in a bowl of water, then rinse off the dirty water and keep them in the fridge. Now they are as alive as any fresh food and need to be preserved cold. You can keep them in water, and they will last 3-4 days in the fridge.

2. **Mixed-up Seed Bread DRY**

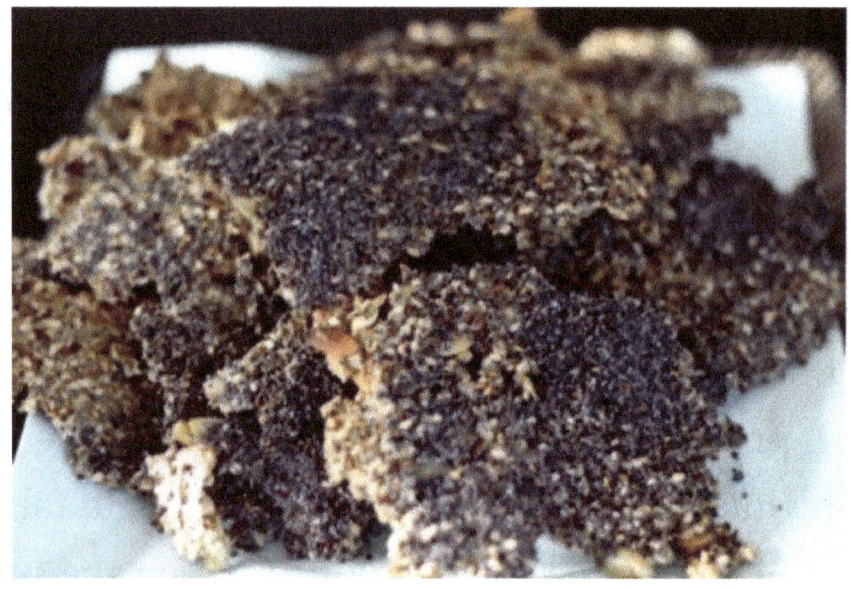

Ingredients (equal amounts of each)

- Quinoa flakes
- Flax seeds
- Sunflower seeds

- Sesame seeds

- Pumpkin seeds

- 1tbs Coconut fat (optional)

- Water

- Poppy seeds for topping

PROCESS:

Start by preheating the oven to 180C. With this flatbread, it's important to use equal amounts of flakes and seeds, add them mix them all in a bowl with 1tbs of virgin coconut oil (which will make your bread crispy, but this is optional). -Slowly add a little bit of water and start mixing. You need to get the consistency smooth enough so that you can spread the bread onto a baking sheet. -After spreading the mixture onto the sheet, sprinkle poppy seeds on the top and put them in the oven. Let it cook for around 5-10 minutes, depending on the thickness, or until the bread is nice and crisp. Simply you can use any type of seeds for this flatbread, and once you get into your cooking flow, you will have staple favorites. -Remove from the oven, put on a rack to cool off, and enjoy!

3. Flat Bread for Tree Huggers

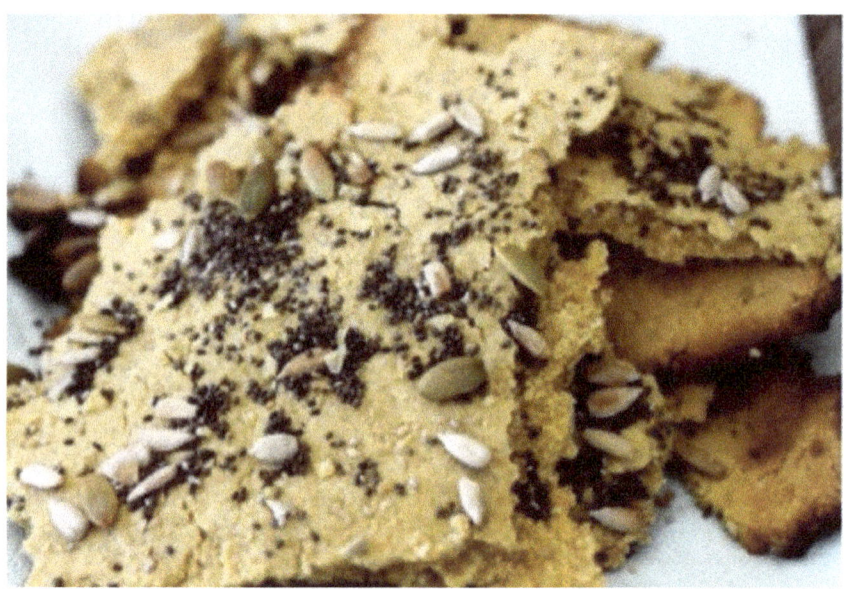

Ingredients

- 150 grams Soy flour
- 150 grams Buckwheat
- 50 grams Quinoa flakes
- ½ tbs of bicarbonate of soda
- One teaspoon of baking powder
- 1tbs Olive oil
- Water
- For Topping (Pumpkin, Poppy and/or Sunflower seeds)

PROCESS:

Start by preheating the oven to 180C. Then in a bowl, mix in your flours with 1tbs of olive oil. Just as with the other flatbread recipe, add a little bit of water at a time and start mixing slowly until you get a nice, smooth, porridge-like consistency. -For those of you who have been at Olive, you know that the consistency needs to be porridge. This means it needs to be smooth enough so that you can spread the bread onto a silicone baking sheet, which once you have done, top it off with the different seeds.

Let it cook for around 5-10 minutes, depending on the thickness, or until the bread is cooked. If you want to have softer bread, remove it from the oven earlier.

This flatbread is great with many of the dishes in the book, especially the curry!

4. **Quinoa Yogi-Power Porridge (serves 4)**

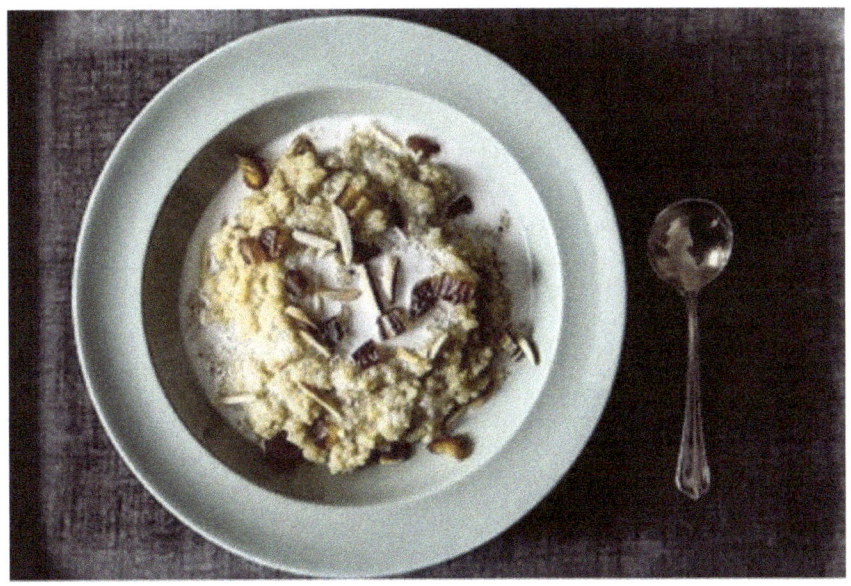

Ingredients:

- 20 grams of Almonds
- 100 grams of Quinoa
- 100 grams of Buckwheat
- 100 grams of water (or as much as is needed)
- 150 grams of Almond milk or Soy milk
- Two tbs of agave
- A pinch of Salt
- 1 Cinnamon stick
- A few pitted Dates

PROCESS:

Rinse the quinoa and buckwheat the usage of a sieve until the rinse water runs out. Put the rinsed water and grains in a pan and boil the mix for a couple of minutes. Remove it from the stove and rinse once more. We try this to dispose of the sour enzymes, which can be hard to digest for people with sensitive stomachs. Put the buckwheat and quinoa back inside the pan and add some of the agave syrup, sea salt, cinnamon, soy or almond milk, and water and bring to a boil. After it is boiling, reduce the heat until the quinoa & buckwheat are fluffy, and all the liquid has been absorbed (about 15-20 mins). Turn off the heat and fluff lightly with a fork. Remove the cinnamon stick. Quickly, before it receives cold, divide the porridge into bowls. Top each with about two tablespoons of soy/ almond milk, along with some almond slivers.

5. Chia Seed Pudding (Serves 4-6)

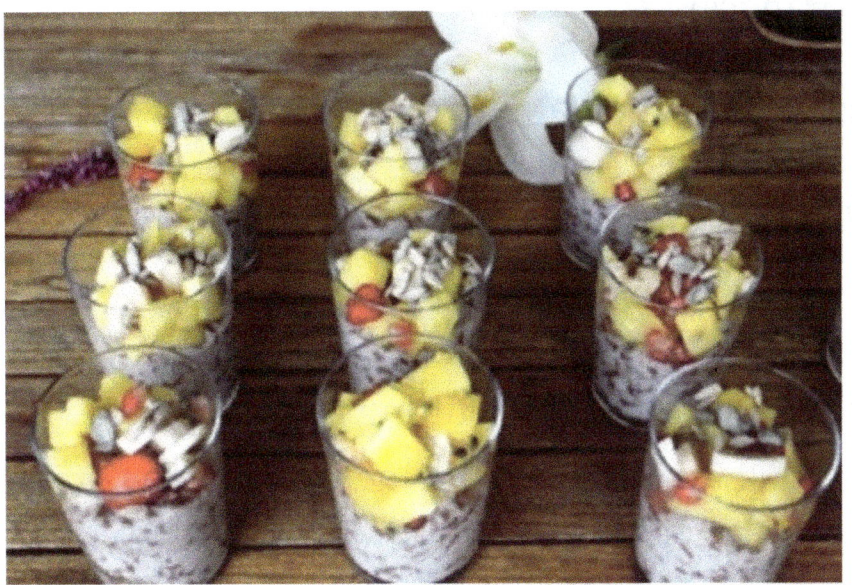

Ingredients

For the pudding:

- 300 grams of Almond milk

- 3tbs of Maple syrup

- One teaspoon of Vanilla bean, seeds scraped

- 1/4 teaspoon of Cardamom

- 50 grams of Chia seeds (you can add a little more if you like the pudding to be thicker)

For the honey-poached Clementine:

- 3 Clementine's, peeled and segments separated

- 100 grams of water

- Half cup of fresh Orange juice (this can be from clementine or regular oranges)

- One teaspoon of Vanilla

- 3tbs of honey

PROCESS:

Make the chia seed pudding by putting all the ingredients in a medium-sized mixing bowl and stir to combine everything. Transfer to another dish, cover, and place in the refrigerator overnight (or for a minimum of three hours). Make the clementine by placing the water, orange juice, vanilla, and honey in a small pot and bring to a boil. Lessen the heat and let it simmer for TEN minutes. Add in the clementine and let it simmer for TEN minutes. Remove from the heat and put it into a separate bowl. Spoon the chia seed pudding into bowls, and place the poached clementine on top. Sprinkle a little of the remaining poaching liquid over the pudding. The chia seed pudding will keep for several days in an airtight container in the fridge, but if you are serving it with the clementine, then it is best to poach them right before you are ready to serve.

6. Pancake Domination

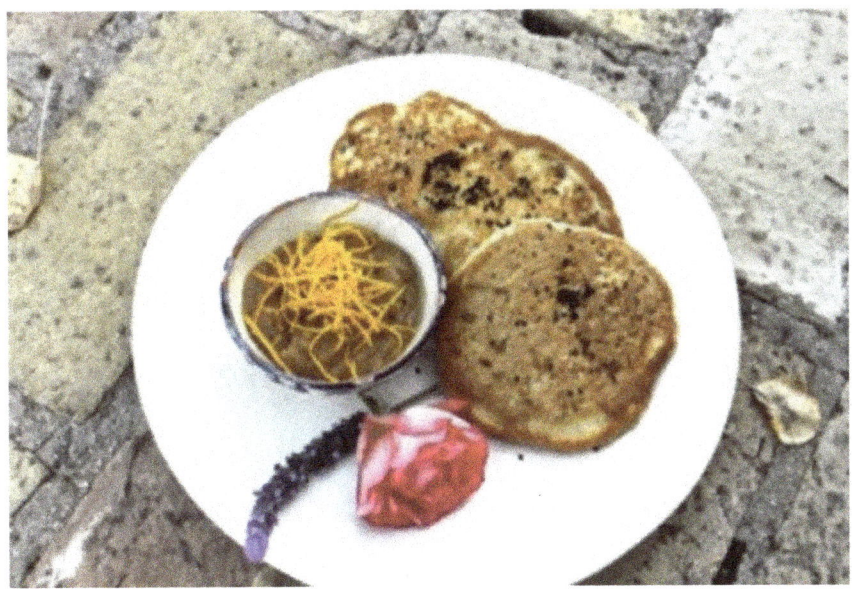

Ingredients

- 1 Flax (1 tablespoon Flaxseed meal + 2tablespoonwaterr for binding)

- Vanilla extract or Vanilla pods

- 100 grams unsweetened Almond milk

- One tablespoon natural salted Peanut butter

- One Tablespoon of Virgin Coconut oil – for cooking

- One tablespoon Agave syrup

- 1tsp Baking powder

- ½tbs of bicarbonate

- A pinch of Salt

- 100 grams Buckwheat flour

- 100 grams Oat flour (If you are celiac, use soy or other gluten-free flours)

PROCESS:

Preheat your pan on the stove. You want the pan's surface to be hot, but not too hot that the oil smokes when it makes contact with the pan's surface. In a large mixing bowl, add your ingredients, flaxseed, and water, and let it sit for a minute or two. Then, add the agave, peanut butter, bicarb, baking powder, whisk, Salt, and vanilla extract. Add whisk and almond milk again until well combined. Next, add 1tsp Baking powder, ½tbs of Bicarbonate, A pinch of Salt, 100 grams Buckwheat flour, 100 grams Oat flour (If you are celiac, use soy or other gluten-free flours), and stir it until it is mixed.

Let the batter rest for FIVE minutes. Lightly grease your pan and pour measurements of the batter onto the pan. There should be enough for SIX pancakes. Flip the pancakes until bubbles appear in the middle and the edges turn a little bit dry. Be careful not to burn them. Cook for ONE-TWO minutes more on the other side and then top with more peanut butter and a light drizzle of agave, or whatever else pleases you. Bananas and other fruits will also go in the mix for taste.

7. Nutty Milks

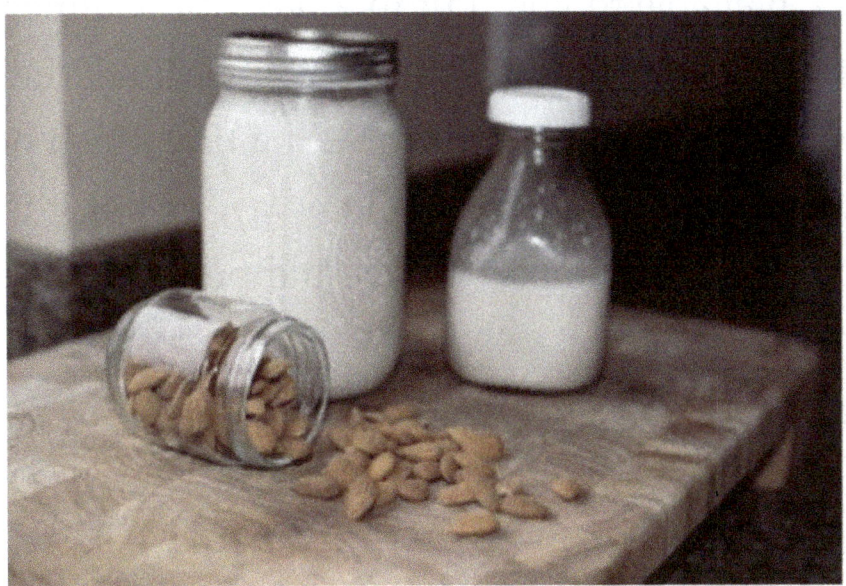

Ingredients:

- 1 liter of filtered water

- Handful of Almonds

- Tiny Pinch of Salt Spice up your Milk

- Cardamom

- Cinnamon

- Vanilla

- Clove

- Nutmeg

You can also Add anything you like

PROCESS:

Pour 1-liter of water in a good blender (we use Vitamix), but you can use any that is available to you. Put in a handful of almonds and blend until the water turns white and milky. You can then either strain the milk or leave it as is, milky and thick. Add a tiny pinch of Salt and any spices. Blend again and enjoy it straight away, or put it in the fridge to get it nice and cold. Remember to save the pulp for cakes, bread, and stews, to name a few.

8. SMOOTHIES

A refreshing start to your morning. This would also serve as a tasty dessert.

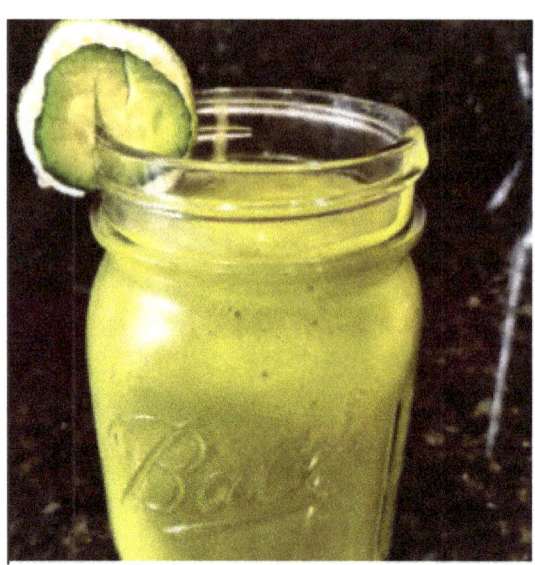

Ingredients

- 1/2 banana (frozen or fresh)
- 1/4 cup frozen pineapple
- 1/4 cup cold or frozen grapes
- One bunch spinach (or other dark green)

Process:

Put the vegetables and fruit in the blender. Add plant-based milk (such as almond, soy, rice, or coconut), water, or juice (with no added sugar) up to 2 cups. Blend well (makes one serving).

9. TOFU SCRAMBLE

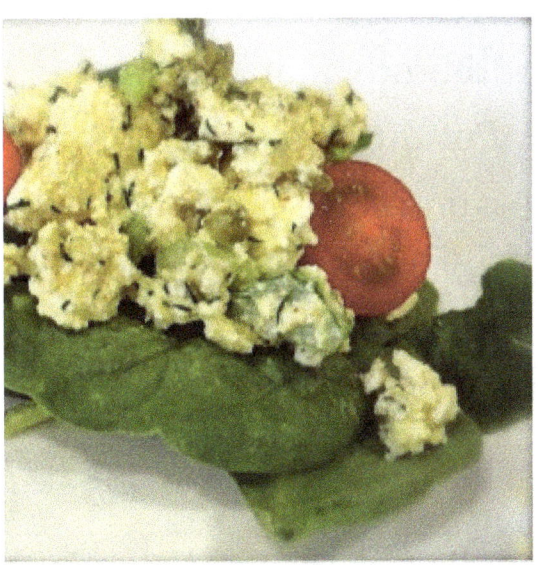

Ingredients

- 1/2 cup vegetable broth
- 1 cup chopped fresh kale
- 1/2 cup onion celery
- 16 oz low-fat tofu, drained crumbled
- 1/2 cup chopped onion
- 1/4 tsp salt
- 1/2 cup chopped bell pepper
- 1/4 tsp pepper

- 1/2 cup chopped carrots
- 1 tsp dried basil

Process

Heat 1/4 cup broth in a pan over medium heat. Put celery, onion, bell pepper, and carrots. Add broth a tablespoon at a time to avoid burning. Cook until it gets soft. Put the remaining 1/4 cup broth and kale. Now cover the pan and cook until kale is wilted. Add tofu. Cook until firm and lightly browned. Add Salt, black pepper, and basil.

10. "FRIED" POTATOES:

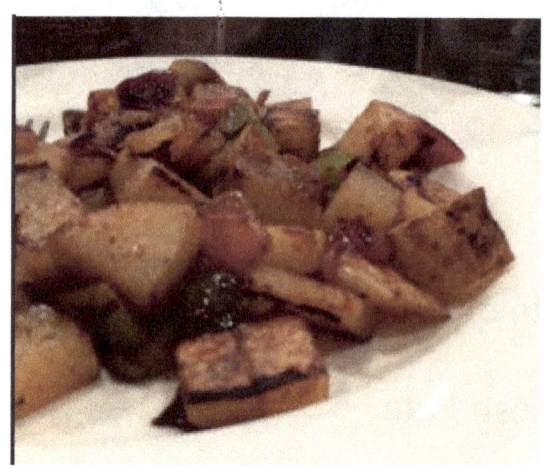

Ingredients:

- One medium onion chopped
- One russet potato chopped
- 1/2-inch cubes
- One garlic clove minced (if desired)

- One jalapeño pepper minced (if desired)
- One green or red bell pepper

Process:

Heat the pan on medium heat and add 1/4 cup of vegetable broth. Add onions and fry until onions are clear. Continue to add broth or water, a tablespoon at a time, as it evaporates. Add peppers and potatoes and cook until done.

11. TROPICAL FRUIT SALAD WITH MINT SAUCE

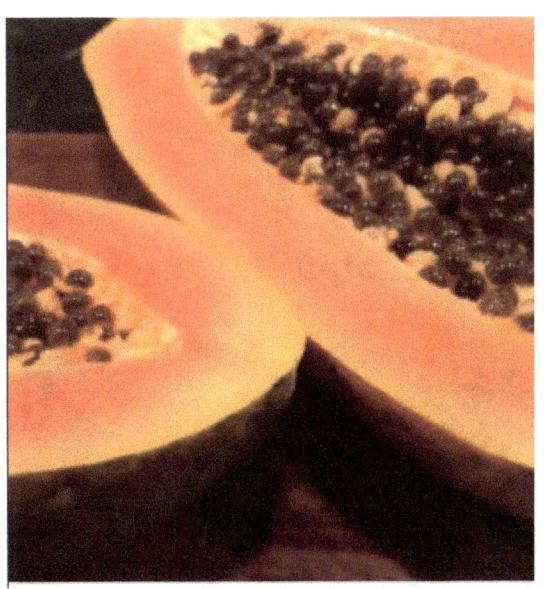

Ingredients

For Papaya Mint Sauce:

Half tablespoon of papaya, peeled, seeded, and coarsely chopped

One Tablespoon of agave nectar

Two tablespoons of fresh lime juice, one and a half tbsp fresh mint

For Salad:

Half papaya, peeled, seeded, and chopped in 1/2-inch cubes

Half pineapple, peeled and chopped in 1/2-inch pieces

Two bananas, peeled and cut into 1/2-inch pieces

Shredded toasted coconut flakes

Shredded toasted coconut flakes

Process:

Puree sauce ingredients until smooth. Cover and refrigerate. Mix fruit in a large bowl, then spoon into bowls and drizzle with mint sauce. Garnish with shredded coconut.

12. Lebanese Roast Ratatouille with Hummus

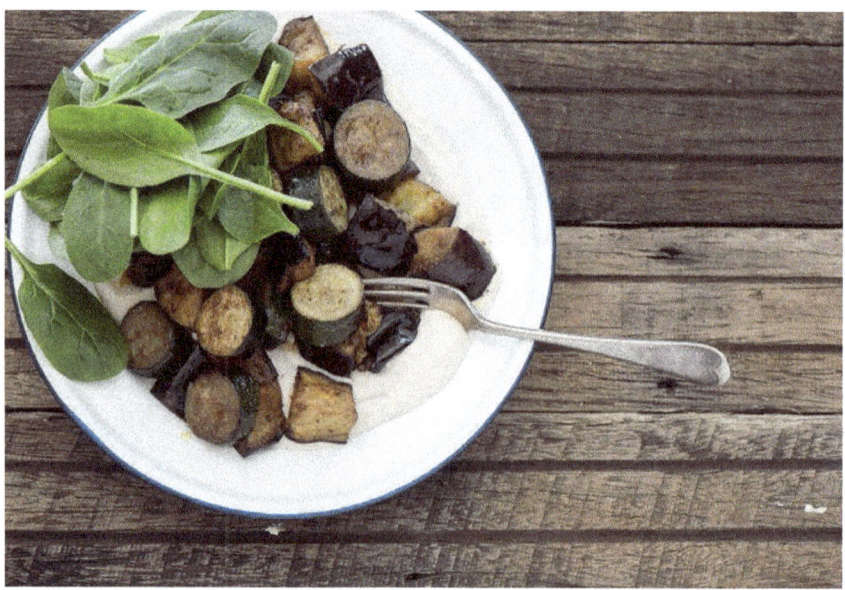

Ingredients:

- Two medium eggplant
- Three small zucchinis
- Two teaspoons Cayenne pepper
- spice blend
- 4-6 tablespoons extra virgin olive oil
- 300g (9oz) hummus
- salad greens, to serve

Process:

Preheat your oven to 480 F. Chop zucchini and eggplant into 2.5cm chunks (1 inch). Toss zucchini, eggplant, oil, and spices in a roasting pan. Sprinkle with Salt. Roast for 25-30 minutes, stirring about halfway or until zucchini and eggplant are well cooked and starting to brown. Divide hummus between 2 plates. Top with roast veg and salad leaves.

13. Coconut Berry Swirl

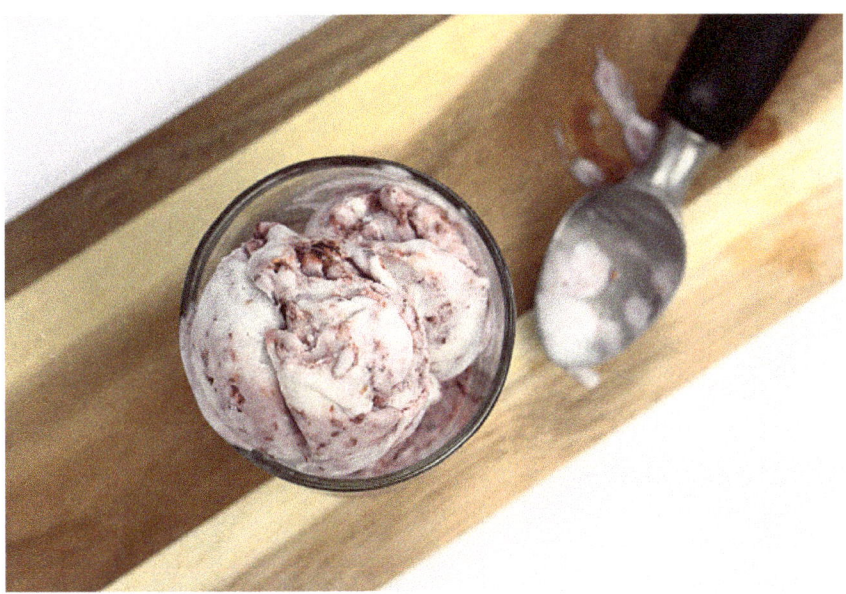

Ingredients:

- Two handfuls berries
- Two large scoops of coconut yogurt

Process:

Take a fork and mash berries in it. Scoop yogurt into two bowls, then swirl your berry mash through the coconut.

14. BANANA BREAD

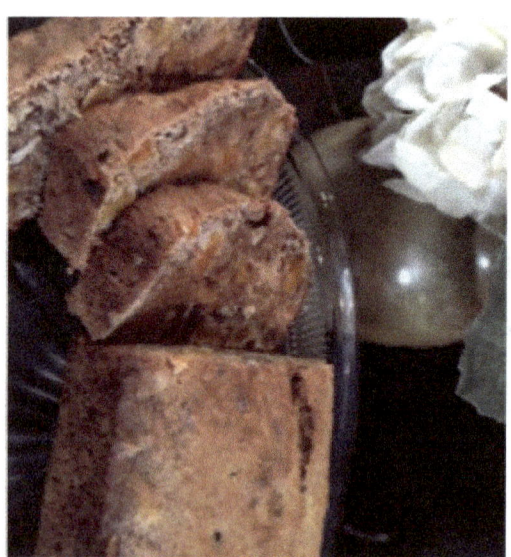

Ingredients:

- 1 cup whole wheat flour
- 1 cup ripe banana (about 2)
- 1 cup whole grain oat flour
- 1/2 cup maple syrup
- 1 tsp baking soda
- 1/3 cup unsweetened applesauce

- 1/2 tsp salt
- 1/4 cup plant-based milk
- 2 tsp pumpkin pie spice
- 1 cup chopped dried apricots
- 1/2 cup chopped pecans
- 1/4 cup toasted coconut flakes

Process:

Preheat the oven to 350 degrees. Spray 9 x 4-inch loaf pan with cooking spray. In a bowl, mix flour, soda, Salt, and spice and mix well. In a mixing bowl, mix banana, syrup, applesauce, and milk. Blend well. Mix Ingredients. Add apricots, pecans, and coconut flakes. Pour mixture into the pan. Bake for 60-70 minutes until the toothpick in the middle comes out clean.

Lunch

15.   A "WHAT" SALAD SANDWICH

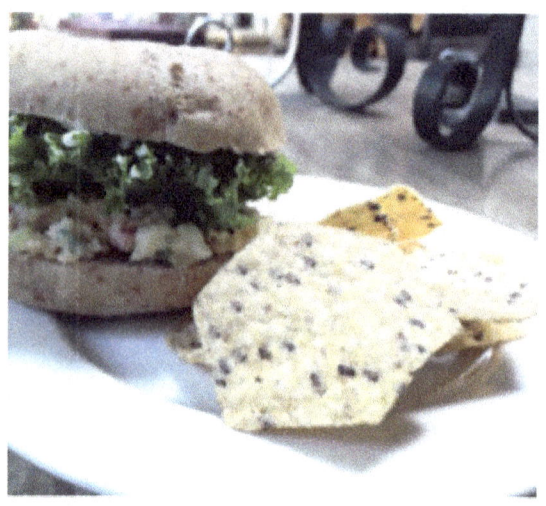

Ingredients:

- 1.15 oz can chickpeas
- One garlic clove
- Two stalks of celery, finely chopped
- 1 1/2 tablespoon of Yellow Mustard
- Three green onions, thinly sliced
- One and a half - 3 tsp lemon juice
- 1/4 cup finely chopped dill pickle
- Half tablespoon salts
- Half cup finely chopped red bell pepper
- Freshly ground black pepper

- 2 tbsp vegan mayonnaise, such as Vegenaise

Process:

In a food processor, lightly chop chickpeas into a flaky texture (you can use a potato masher too). Stir in celery, peppers, pickles, green onions, Garlic, and mayonnaise until combined. Stir in Mustard and season with salt, pepper, and lemon juice to taste. Serve with sprout bagel, lettuce wrap, or whole wheat crackers.

16. GRILLED PORTOBELLO MUSHROOM AND QUINOA SALAD

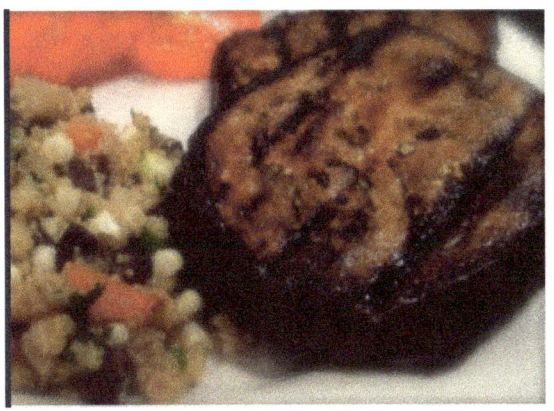

For marination:

Ingredients:

- 3 tbsp soy sauce,
- 3 tbsp brown rice syrup,
- Three cloves minced garlic

- 1 tbsp grated ginger

Process:

Marinate your mushrooms in 3 tbsp soy sauce, 3 tbsp brown rice syrup, three cloves minced Garlic, and 1 tbsp grated ginger for about an hour, then throw on the grill.

For salad

Ingredients:

- two and a half cups cooked quinoa
- two cups of corn,
- one bell pepper chopped,
- 1/2 small red onion
- 2 cups black peans,
- 1 cup cilantro chopped,
- Six green onions sliced
- One jalapeño

Process:

The salad is made by combining 2 1/2 cups cooked quinoa, 2 cups of corn, one bell pepper chopped, half small red onion diced, 2 cups black beans, 1 cup cilantro chopped, six green onions sliced, and one jalapeño pepper minced (if desired). Top with the juice of 2 limes.

17. Andalusian Tomato Salad

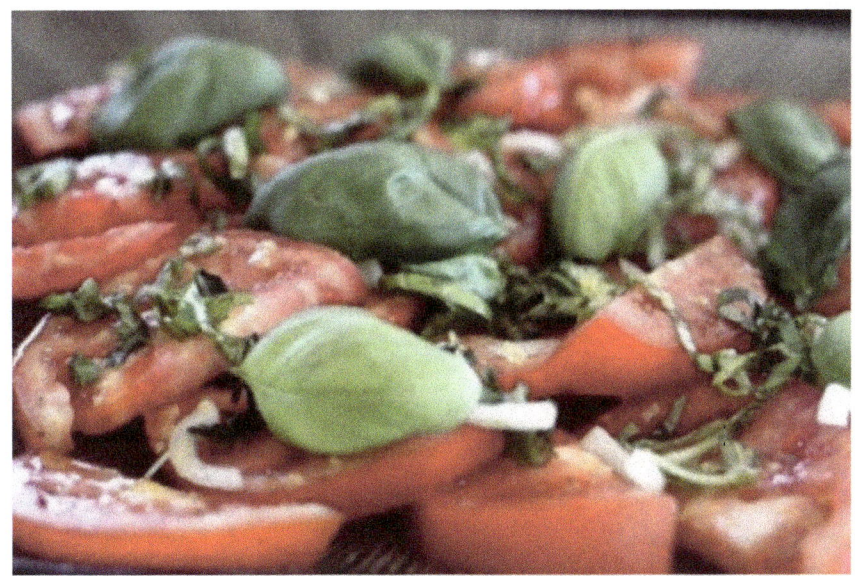

Ingredients

- 3-4 Big Juicy Tomatoes
- 2-3 Spring Onions

Basil for dressing & Garnish

- Olive oil
- Orange juice (from 1 real orange)
- Lemon juice (from 1 real lemon)
- One grated Garlic
- Pinch of Salt & Pepper

Process:

Chop your tomatoes in whatever shape you think looks nice, along with your spring onions. Arrange beautifully on a big plate, drizzle olive oil, squeeze the juice of your real lemon, and orange on top of the tomatoes. Grate your garlic clove and massage it into your tomatoes. Sprinkle on the spring onions, and top it off with your fresh basil leaves and a pinch of salt & pepper.

18.   Green Salad Supremacy

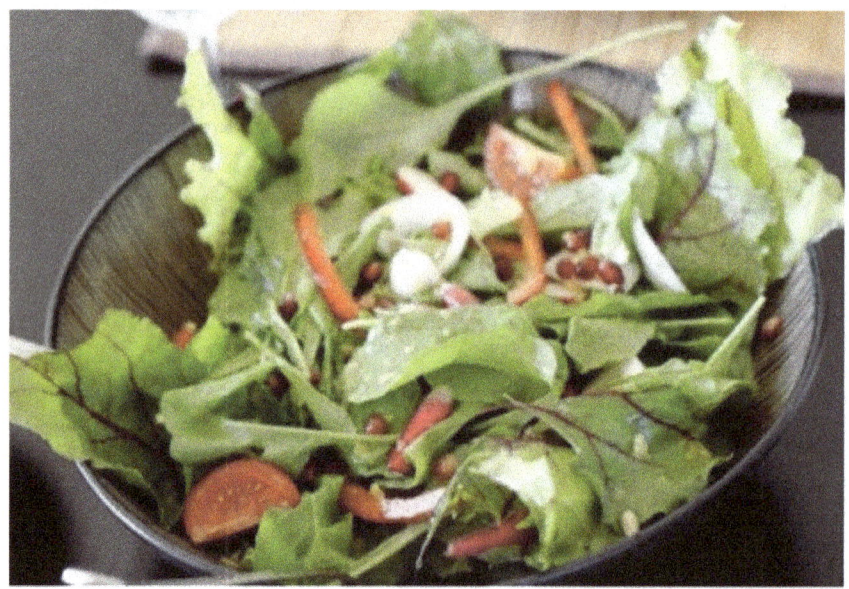

Ingredients:

- Mixed leaves
- Beetroot leaves
- Salad onion
- Red peppers
- Radishes
- Pomegranate seeds
- Tomatoes
- Olive oil

- Lemon juice

- Salt & Pepper

- Chopped chives

- Dijon mustard

- Agave syrup

PROCESS:

Start off with your dressing: chop the spring onions and put them into a bowl. Add olive oil, lemon juice, Dijon mustard, agave, and a pinch of salt & pepper, and then mix all together. Voila, it's ready! The amount of ingredients depends on how much dressing you would like. Sometimes it's a good idea to make a big batch and keep it in the fridge. Whether it's sweeter, tangier, or saltier depends on how you want it. Taste your way toward the right dressing for you. Chop up all your greens and arrange them nicely in a bowl or on a big plate, and drizzle the dressing on top! Always drizzle the dressing on just before serving and never, ever mix the salad after pouring the dressing on top! Within seconds your leaves will get heavy & soggy.

19. Orange & Coriander Kindness

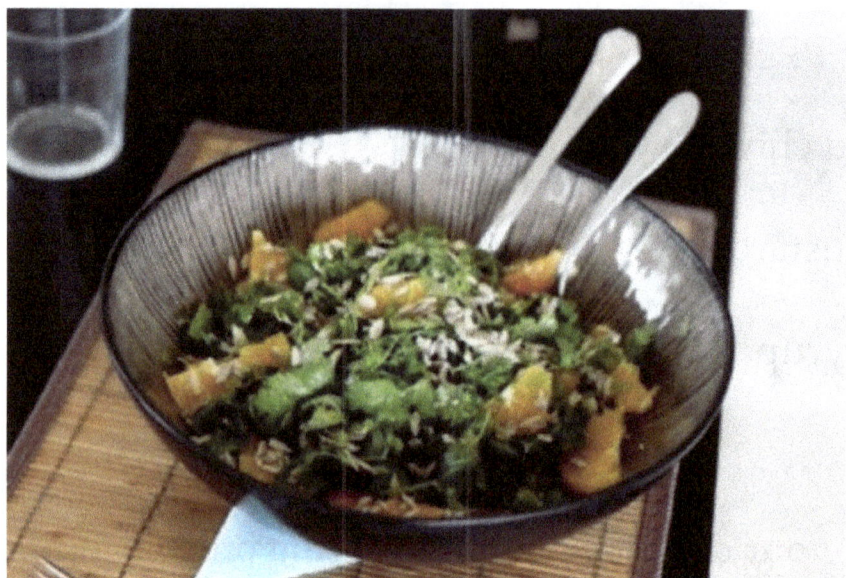

Ingredients

- Lots of fresh Coriander
- 1 Orange
- Lightly toasted Sunflower seeds

Tamari Dressing

- Olive oil (2tbs)
- Tamari
- Lemon juice
- Grated ginger
- Grated Garlic

PROCESS

If you have a bunch of coriander, pick off all the leaves and put them in a salad bowl. Save the stalks for stir-fries, curries, or as a flavor for a paste. Always try and use every part of a vegetable! Cut the orange into small pieces and scatter it around the leaves. Dress the salad with the dressing made by mixing olive oil, Tamari, lemon juice, grated ginger, and Garlic. It's good to keep this dressing handy in the fridge because it can be used for many different dishes or even as a marinade. Top off the salad with your lightly toasted sunflower seeds. This salad is fantastic with spicy foods. The sweetness of the orange cuts through any spice and adds freshness from the coriander leaves.

20. **Cozy Winter Salad**

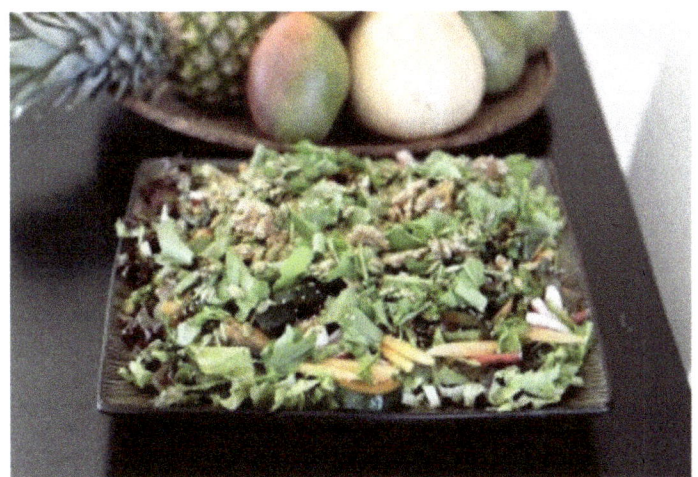

Ingredients:

The base of the Salad:

- 3-4 Types of lettuce leaves
- Rocket & Carrot shoots
- Fresh and crisp Garnish

Top of the salad (stir Fried with Tamari):

- Zucchini
- Shallots/Spring Onions
- Green peppers
- Asparagus
- Mushrooms
- French Beans
- Spring onion tops (green part)

Fresh & Crisp:

- Baby Carrots/or regular ones (keep the shoots for decoration)
- Radishes
- Roots of Spring onion (white part) Toasted:
- Walnuts
- Pumpkin Seeds
- Sesame Seeds

Garlic & Mustard infused Dressing

- 100 grams of Olive oil
- One clove of Garlic

- 1tbs Mustard seeds

- Juice of 1 Lemon

- Pinch of Salt & Pepper

Process:

Start by washing and prepping all your veggies and putting them into piles of fresh and crisp, stir-fried & base. The fresh & crisp vegetables you can put in a bowl with water and store in the fridge until you need to use them. Chop your stir-fried pile and put it to one side, and do the same with your lettuce base. We like to use red & green Lolo lettuce, baby gem, spinach, or any other type of green leaf. With this recipe, you want to pre-prepare your dressing. Start off by gently heating the olive oil with finely chopped Garlic & mustard seeds. Take it off the heat when the garlic and mustard seeds are sizzling. Then add the lemon juice, salt, pepper, and leave to one side. The longer the ingredients marry, the better. In a small pan, toast your nuts. We would use a pinch of each; again, amounts depend on taste and the size of the salad. At this stage, we are ready to put everything together! Start off by arranging the base (greens) on a beautiful platter with different types of green leaves. Stir-fry main vegetables with a splash of Tamari until nice and soft. Arrange on top of your greens, then add your fresh & crisp vegetables followed by rocket & carrot shoots. Drizzle the garlic mustard seed dressing on top just before serving! This recipe might look daunting at first, but as long as you do all your prep beforehand, it's only a matter of putting the ingredients together. It's a great winter warmer especially considering that you don't always feel like having a cold salad on a cold rainy day.

21. Crispy Broccolini & Chickpeas with Cashew 'Ricotta'

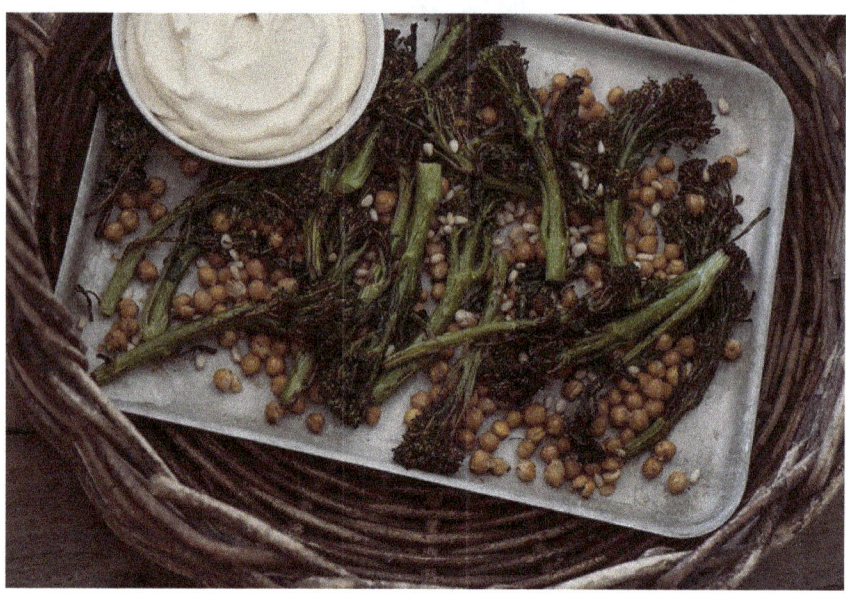

Ingredients

- One Can chickpeas (400g / 14oz), drained.

- Two bunches of broccolini 200g (7oz) cashews

- Four tablespoons lemon juice + extra to serve

- Four tablespoons extra virgin olive oil

- handful pine nuts (optional)

Process:

Preheat your oven to 250C (480F) – place broccolini and chickpeas on a baking tray. Drizzle generously with oil and put it in the oven for 20-25 minutes. While the broccolini and chickpeas are cooking, cover cashews with boiling water and stand for a few minutes—drain cashews and place them in your food processor or blender. Add half cup water, lots of salt, and four tablespoons of lemon juice. Stir till you've got a smooth, creamy sauce, scraping the sides down a few times. Give it at least 5 minutes. Gradually sprinkle in four tablespoons of extra virgin olive oil. Taste and season with lemon and more salt, as per your own taste. When the broccolini stems are cooked perfectly, and their edges are nice and crispy, sprinkle over some pine nuts (if using) and put them back in the oven for a minute or two. Serve your roast with a little extra lemon juice squeezed over and cashew sauce on the side.

22.   Quick Chickpea Curry

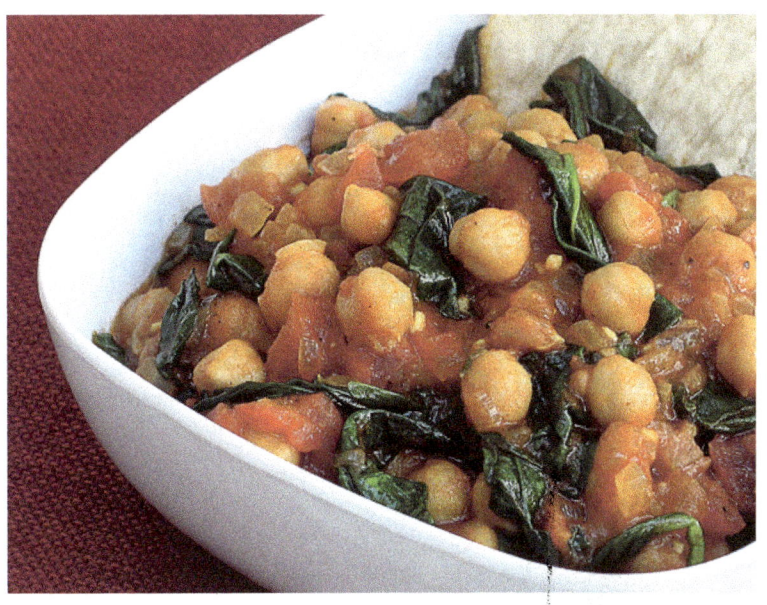

Ingredients

- Two red onions, Sliced in Half
- 3-4 teaspoons curry powder
- One can of tomatoes (400g / 14oz)

- 400g (14oz) cooked chickpeas (or two cans)
- One bag of baby spinach

Process:

Heat a small quantity of olive oil in a pan on medium heat. Add red onions, cover, and cook until the onion is soft but not browned. Stir every now and then. It will take about 5-10 minutes. Add curry powder and let it cook for about 30 seconds, then add the chickpeas and tomatoes. Simmer covered for 6-10 minutes or until everything is piping hot. Taste and season with salt, pepper, and extra curry powder if needed. Serve on a bed of baby spinach.

23. Spiced Chickpeas with Cauli Mash

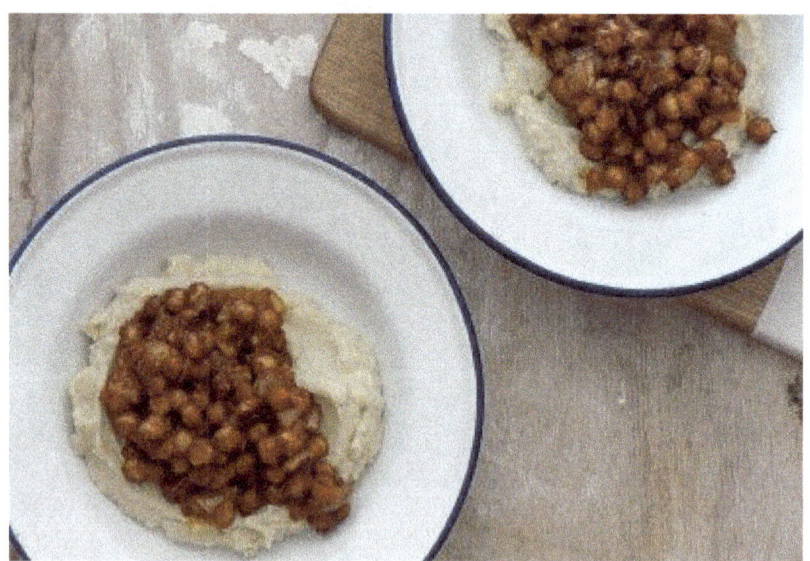

Ingredients

- 1/2 medium cauliflower, chopped
- Four tablespoons coconut oil

- One onion, chopped

- One teaspoon Cayenne pepper

- One can chickpea (400g / 14oz), drained.

- Four tablespoons tomato paste

Process:

Bring 1in(2cm) water to boil in a medium pan. Put cauli and simmer covered for 8-15 minutes or until cauli is really tender. (add more water as needed-Be careful not to let it dry out and burn). Meanwhile, melt 1/2 of the coconut oil in a small pan. Cook onion on medium heat until soft but not browned, about 5-10 minutes. When the onion is soft, add the chickpeas, tomato, and spice. Stir well and bring to a simmer. Remove from the heat, taste, and season with pepper and salt. When the cauli is drained, cooked, and return to the pan, you cooked it in with the remaining coconut oil. Pour with a stick blender or mash well with a fork. Serve spiced chickpeas on a bed of cauli mash.

24. Red Lentils with Tomato & Spinach

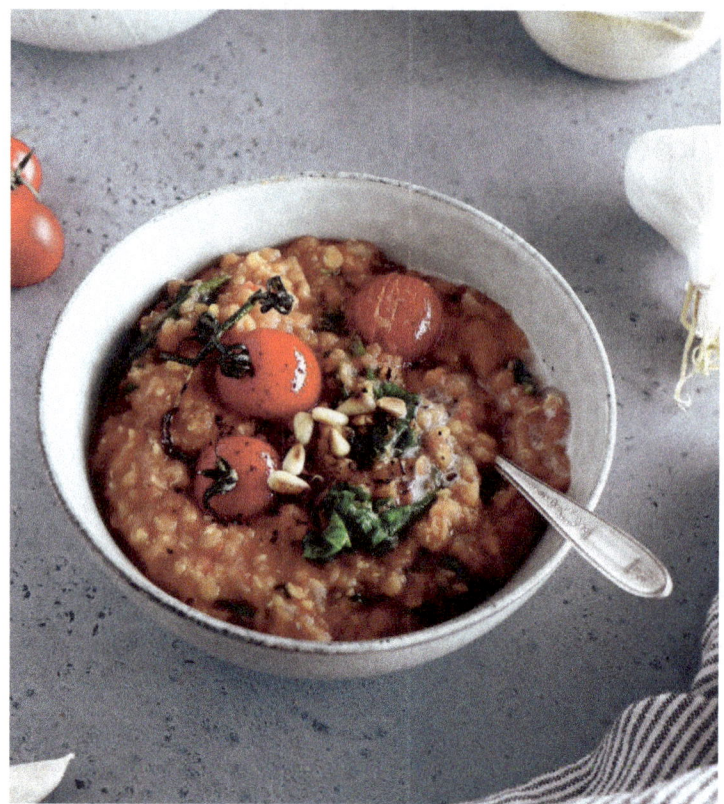

Ingredients:

- Two cloves garlic, peeled & finely sliced

- 150g (5oz) red lentils

- Three tablespoons tomato paste

- One box frozen spinach (approx 250g / 9oz) OR

- One bag of baby spinach leaves

- One handful almonds, optional

Process:

Heat two tablespoons olive oil for 2-3 minutes in a large pan or skillet. Cook garlic over high heat for about 30 seconds or until starting to brown. Add lentils, frozen spinach (if using), tomato paste, and 1 1/2 cups water. Simmer for about 8 minutes or until lentils are just cooked, but still al dente. Add almonds, and if using baby spinach, add it now. Stir until the spinach is just wilted. Taste, season, and serve.

25.	Zen Habits Three-Bean Veggie Chili

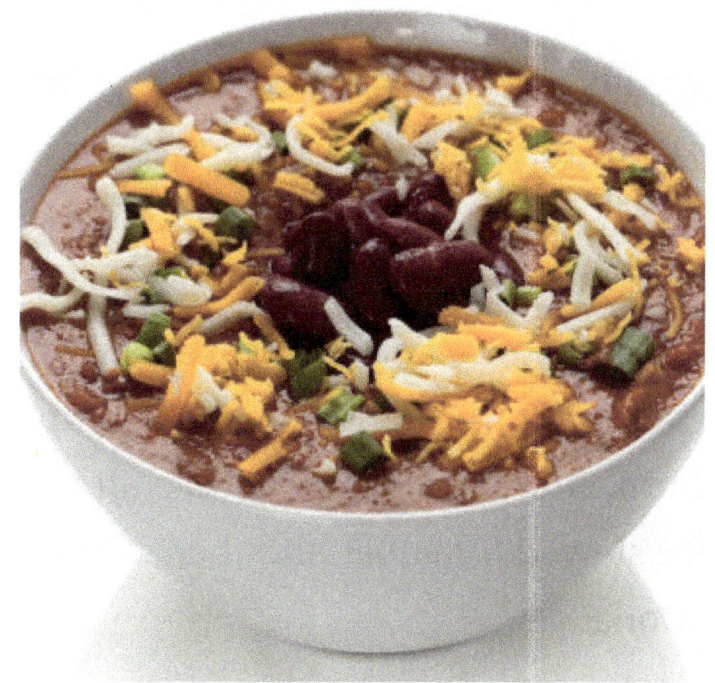

Ingredients

- One package Yves Meatless Ground Round (or any vegan ground beef replacement) --optional

- One 14.5 oz. can each: black beans, pinto beans, and kidney beans

- One 14.5 oz. can corn

- One 29 oz. can each: tomatoes sauce & stewed tomato

- Yellow onion, half, chopped

- Half a green bell pepper, seeded, cored, and diced

- 3-4 cloves garlic, diced (depending on how much you like Garlic)

- salt, Black pepper, chili powder to taste

- Olive oil

Process

Chop the veggies first because the cooking will go fast. On medium-high heat, heat up some olive oil, then saute the onions, then the garlic and bell pepper. Throw in the ground beef replacement (still frozen is fine), and let it brown. Add a liberal amount of black pepper and chili powder and a bit of salt. Now dump in the can of corn and can of beans, one at a time, stirring as you go along, making sure that the bottom doesn't stick and burn. Add black pepper and chili powder. Spice it up nicely. Throw in the stewed tomatoes and then stir, and then dump in the tomato sauce. Done!

Lessen the heat and let it simmer for a while. You can actually eat it right away, or you can simmer it for 20 minutes, an hour, or more. For better flavor, let it simmers for as long as possible. Taste it and spice it as needed. It will taste good if you add a lot of chili powder and black pepper. To crank up the heat, feel free to add your favorite red peppers early on in the cooking process. Also, feel free to add beer to the recipe and let it simmer a bit to soak into the chili. Serve with good bread, brown rice, or blue corn chips. Enjoy!

26.   Gentle Lentils

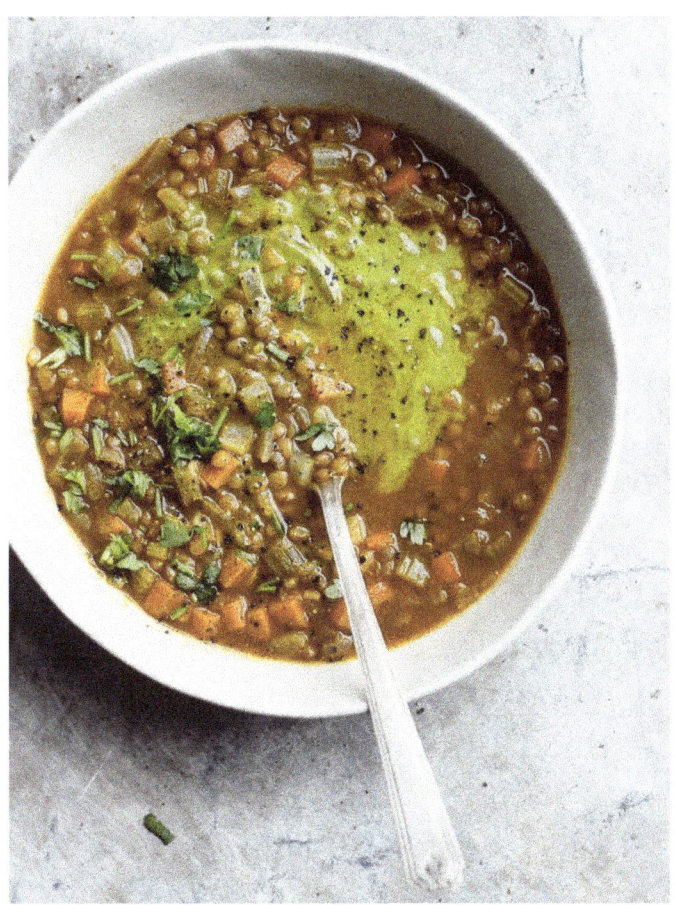

Ingredients

- Pre-soaked/cooked red lentils

- 1 Onion

- 1 Garlic clove

- 2tbs of Coconut cream

- 2tbs Tomato paste

- Olive oil

- Fenugreek seed

- Red sweet Paprika powder

- Salt & Pepper

Process:

Chop the onion in half-moon shapes along with your Garlic, and fry off with some olive oil. Add fenugreek seeds and sweet paprika powder and fry until everything is nice and soft. Then add your pre-cooked red lentils, tomato paste, and a pinch of salt & pepper. Mix it well until it reaches a creamy consistency. At that point, add the coconut cream to bring together the dish nicely and add that extra creaminess! Garnish with coriander or fresh parsley.

27. Spiced Lentils with Hummus

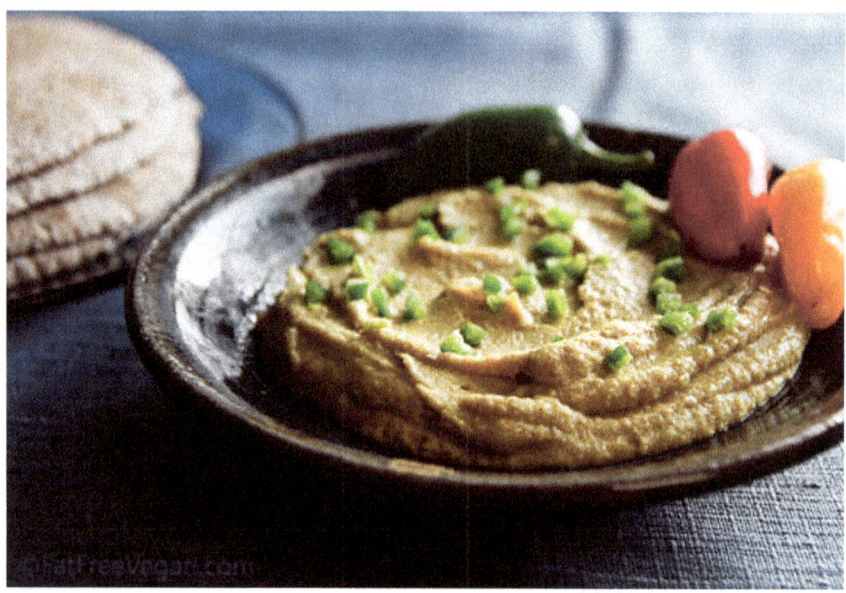

Ingredients

- 200g (7oz) dried puy (or French-style green) lentils

- One onion, chopped

- Two teaspoons Cayenne pepper
- Eight tablespoons hummus
- One bag of baby spinach, to serve

Process:

Bring a pot of medium size put water to a boil in it. Add lentils and simmer until tender, about 15-20 minutes. Meanwhile, heat a little oil on medium heat in a frying pan. Cook onion for 5-10 minutes or until soft. When the lentils are cooked, drain and add lentils and spice to the onions. Cook for about another couple of minutes until everything is warm. Taste. Season. Serve spiced lentils on a bed of hummus with baby spinach on top.

28. CHILI

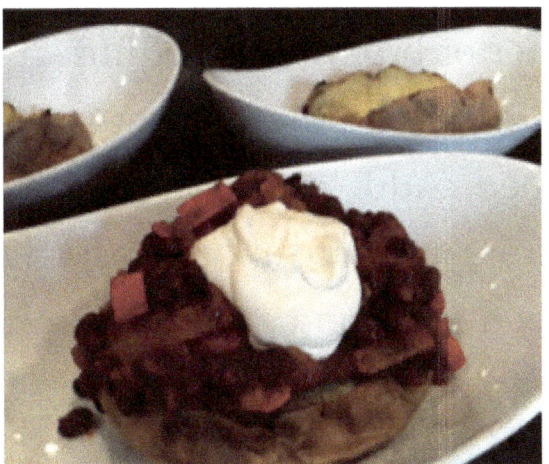

Ingredients:

- One medium onion chopped
- 2.15 oz can black beans

- Two garlic cloves, minced
- 1.15 oz can tomato sauce
- 2 cups mushrooms, sliced
- One green or red bell pepper, chopped
- 1/2 cup golden raisins
- 1 tbsp chile powder
- 1 tsp cumin
- 2 tsp smoked paprika
- 1 tsp cinnamon

Process:

Sauté onion (with water or broth) in a medium-sized pan for 2 minutes. Add Garlic and cook for 1-2 minutes. Put mushrooms and bell peppers and cook until softened. Add spice mixture and cook until fragrant. Add black beans and tomato sauce and cook for 10 minutes until flavors incorporate. Add golden raisin and cook a few more minutes.

Soups

29. Clear Vegetable Soup

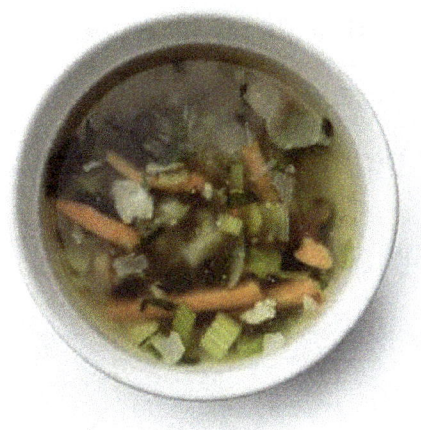

Ingredients:

- 1 cup finely chopped broccoli
- 1 cup, finely chopped carrot
- 1 cup, finely chopped capsicum
- 1 cup, finely chopped green peas
- Six cloves, finely chopped garlic
- 1, peeled, finely chopped onions
- Salt as per taste
- Black pepper powder as per taste
- 2 1/2 cups water
- 1 tsp oil

Process:

Heat oil in a medium pan on a high flame. Now, fry onion and garlic until both turn golden. Then, add all the vegetables and fry for 3-5 minutes. Add some water and allow the mixture to come to a boil. Put the lid onto the pan and then allow the vegetables to cook on low-medium flame. Sprinkle pepper and salt as per taste. Serve hot.

30. **Cauliflower Soup**

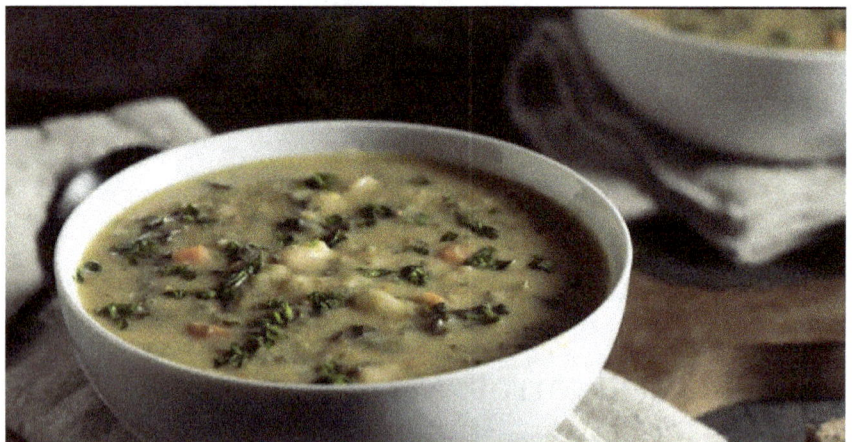

Ingredients

- Cauliflower florets
- Chopped onion
- Chopped potatoes
- Olive oil
- Garlic cloves
- Vegan Cream
- Vegetable stock

Process

In a pan, fry onion and garlic and add cauliflower florets and potato. Add vegetable stock and boil. Add Vegan cream and cook until you get a creamy texture. Serve hot.

31. Moroccan sweet potato lentil

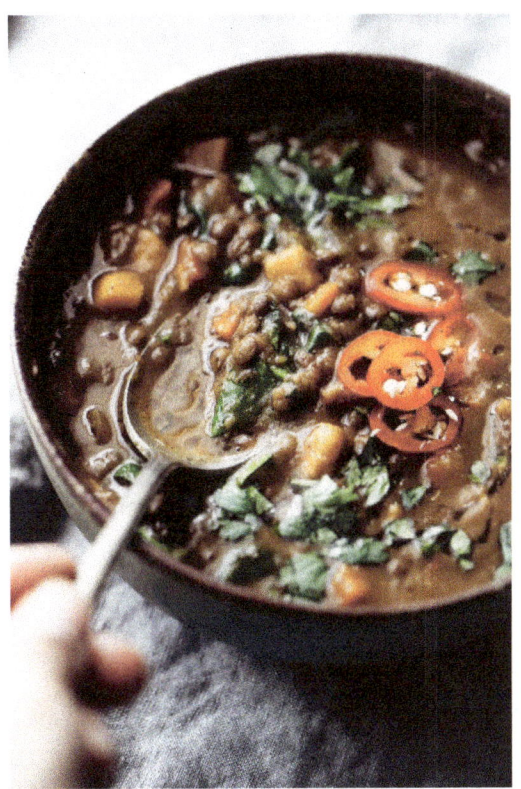

Ingredients

- 1 lb sweet potatoes,
- 1 cup carrots,
- 1 cup onions,
- 1 cup celery,
- One red bell pepper,

- Six cloves garlic,
- 1 ½ cups green or brown lentils,
- 1 ½ teaspoon of coriander
- 1 ½ teaspoon of cumin powder
- One teaspoon of curry powder
- ½ teaspoon of smoked paprika
- ½ teaspoon of ground cinnamon
- ½ teaspoon of turmeric
- ⅛ teaspoon ground nutmeg
- 6-7 cups low sodium broth(vegetables)
- 2 ½ cups baby spinach,
- ¼ cup lemon juice

Process

Place the celery, carrots, onions, sweet potatoes, spices, garlic, lentils, red bell pepper, and 6 cups of broth into a cooker. Cook on low heat for 5-8 hours or on high heat for 3-6 hours. Check the lentils if it cooked enough. If your lentils have been inside the pantry for some time, notice that they bit longer to cook through. Take a blendder and put 1/2 of the soup in it along with add a little more broth (half of the cup or so) and blend until smooth. Add the puree back into the cooker. Stir in the lemon juice and baby spinach . Cover the cooker, unplug it, and allow the ingredients to just hang out for 20-30 minutes or so until the spinach sits down. Season with pepper, salt, and curry powder to taste as desired. Thin with additional broth to desired consistency. Serve warm with whipped greek yogurt, fried pita bread, and tons of fresh herbs (parsley or cilantro) on top.

32. **Mushroom Soup**

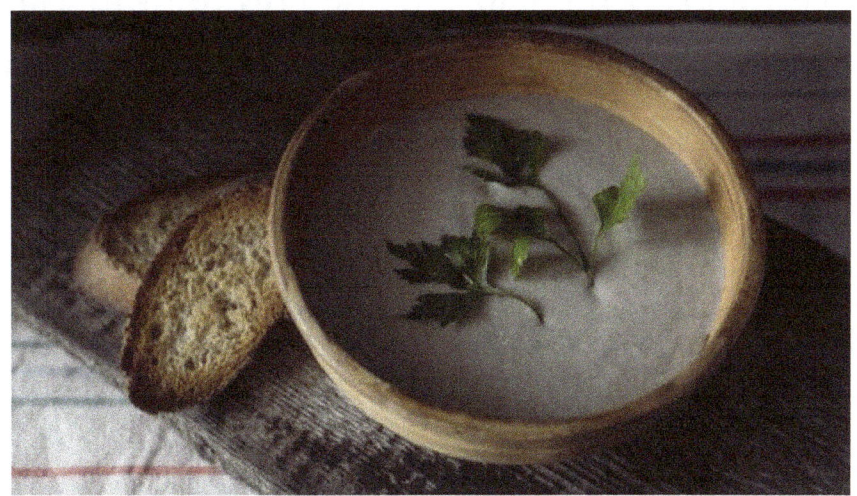

Ingredients:

- 1 cup chopped button mushrooms
- One teaspoon cornflour (dipped in 1/4 teaspoon Hemp milk)
- One sliced small-sized onion
- Salt as per taste
- 1 cup milk of any nuts
- Black pepper as per taste
- 2 cups water

Process:

Add mushrooms and milk to a pan and cook them until mushrooms become soft. Allow it to cool. Once it is cooled, take a blender and make its semi-smooth paste. Now, roast onions in a pan on medium flame until golden. Sprinkle water when required. Remove from pan and keep aside. Then, take the ground paste and mix it with water in a pan; let simmer for 3-5 minutes. Now boil salt and cornflour in a small pan. Now, lower the flame and cook until the mixture turns creamy and thick. Serve hot.

33. Turmeric Tomato Detox Soup

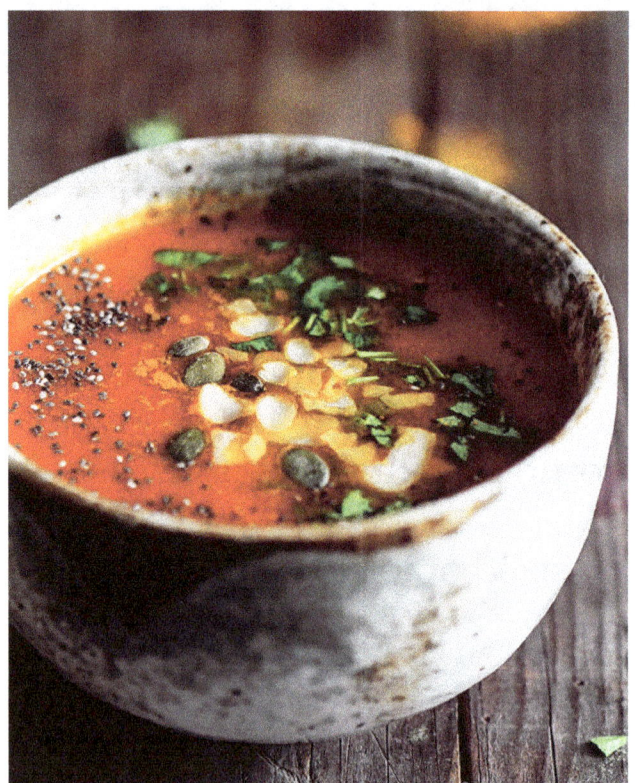

Ingredients

- 5 oz cherry tomatoes

- One can diced tomatoes with their sauce
- ½ cup low-sodium vegetable stock
- One small onion, finely diced
- Two garlic cloves, minced
- 2 tsp turmeric powder
- 1 tsp coconut oil
- ½ tsp sea salt
- 1 tsp dried basil
- 1 tbsp apple cider vinegar
- Freshly ground black pepper
- Mixed seeds and nuts to garnish

Process:

In a small pan, heat coconut oil, then saute the garlic and onion for 1-2 minutes. Put cherry tomatoes and turmeric in a pan and cook them until the tomatoes soften and leave their juices. Add the vegetable stock, tomato can, basil, and apple cider vinegar in a pan and let it boil, cover the pan with a lid, and let it boil for 3-5 minutes. Then put it into the blender to obtain a creamy liquid. Season with pepper and salt and serve garnished with mixed seeds and nuts.

34. Instant Pot Lentil Soup

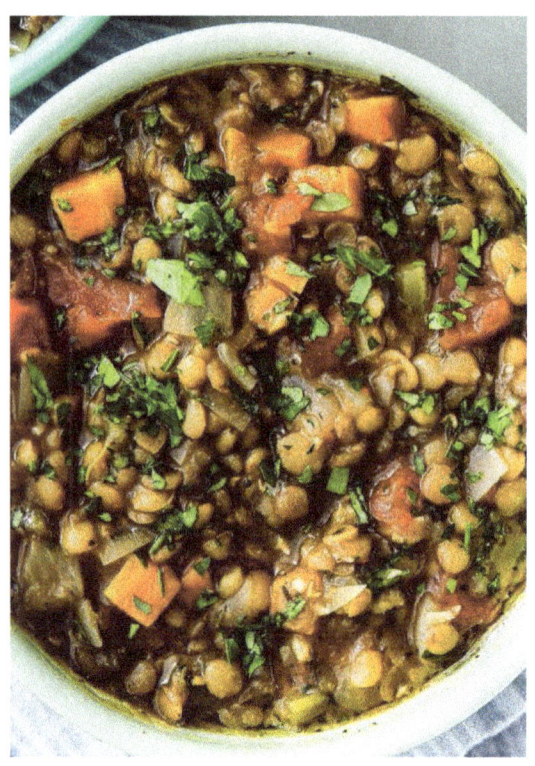

INGREDIENTS

- 1 large onion, chopped
- 1 medium carrot, peeled and chopped
- 2 stalks celery, chopped
- 3 cloves garlic, minced
- 1 1/2 c. green lentils
- 1 (14.5-oz.) can diced tomatoes
- 2 tsp. fresh thyme
- 1 tsp. Italian seasoning

- Kosher salt

- Freshly ground black pepper

- vegetable broth

- baby spinach

- Freshly grated Parmesan, for serving

Process:

To an Instant Pot, add onion, carrot, celery, garlic, lentils, and tomatoes. Add thyme and Italian seasoning and season with salt and pepper. Pour broth over and stir to combine. Set Instant Pot to Manual, High and set for 18 minutes. Once finished, set valve to quick release. Remove lid and stir in spinach. Serve with Parmesan.

35. Veggie-Packed Tomato Soup

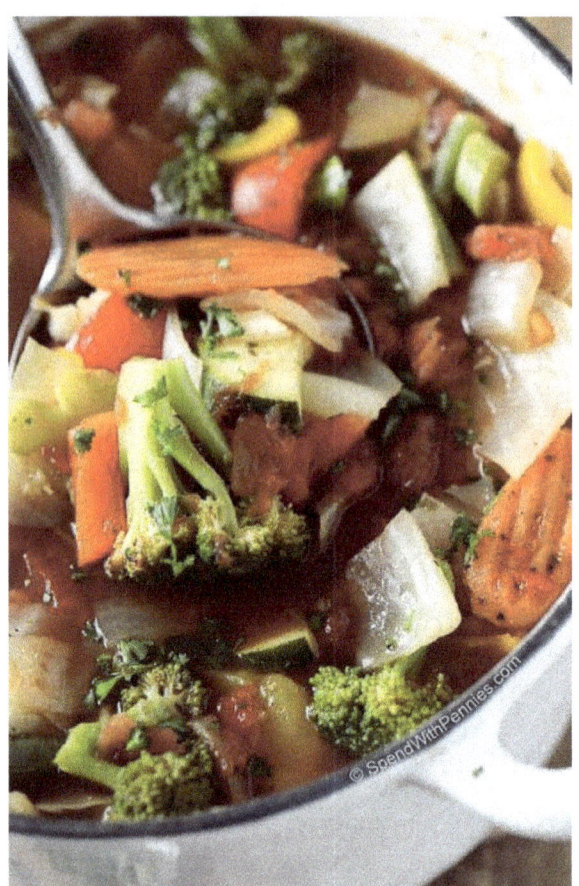

Ingredients

- Vegetable Broth
- Cabbage,
- beans,
- bell peppers,
- tomatoes,
- zucchini,
- broccoli,

- celery
- Carrots,
- potatoes
- sweet potatoes (may need longer to cook)
- Corn

Process

Wash and chop all of your vegetables. Add a touch of oil and fry onion and garlic first for flavor. Add spices or herbs to your liking. Bring broth to a boil, add in vegetables, and allow it to cook until tender. Fry onions and add all ingredients to the slow cooker and cook on high flame for 4-5 hours or low flame for 7-8 hours or until vegetables are tender. Fry onions add all ingredients to the Instant Pot, ensuring you don't go past the max line. Cook on high pressure for 4-8 minutes; naturally, it takes 5 minutes. Cook longer if you prefer softer vegetables.

36. BROCCOLI AND RED LENTIL DETOX SOUP

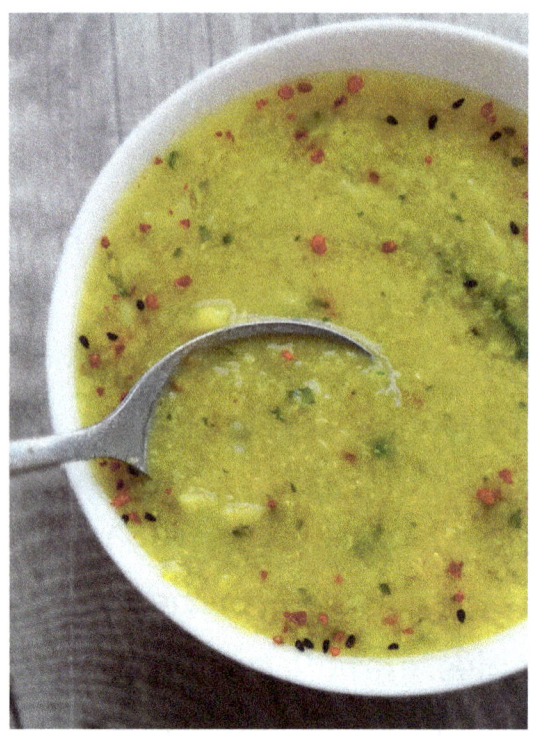

INGREDIENTS

- One medium onion
- One garlic clove
- 1/2 tsp ground cumin
- 1/2 tsp ground turmeric
- 1/2 tsp ground ginger
- 1/3 tsp ground cardamom (optional)
- 1.5 cups broccoli
- 1/2 cup red lentils
- some mint leaves (5-10)

- some cilantro (optional)
- One red chili pepper (optional!)
- Two tablespoon olive oil

Process

Firstly, soak lentils for 30-60mins. Peel onion and garlic, wash vegetables and herbs, chop an onion, broccoli, cilantro (optional), mint leaves, and chili (optional). In a cooking pot, add 1tablespoon of olive oil and fry the garlic and onions at medium flame for about 1-3 mins. Add the spices cumin, optional Cardamom, turmeric, and ginger. Stir and add a little bit of water so that the spices don't burn. Stir again and add chopped lentils, broccoli, half teaspoon of salt, and 3-4 cups of water. Let it cook for 10-15 mins with a lid on the pot until lentils are tender and everything else is cooked. Add mint leaves and optionally cilantro. Turn off heat. With your blend the soup with a hand blender. If you'd like - blend all the way through until smooth (it won't affect the taste, just texture). Add one more tbsp olive oil and stir in. Salt to taste. Add water if too thick (shouldn't be). Optionally: Slice red chili pepper and add at the end. Serve hot, and if you'd like, top with some hot paprika flakes and cumin.

37. Green Detox Soup

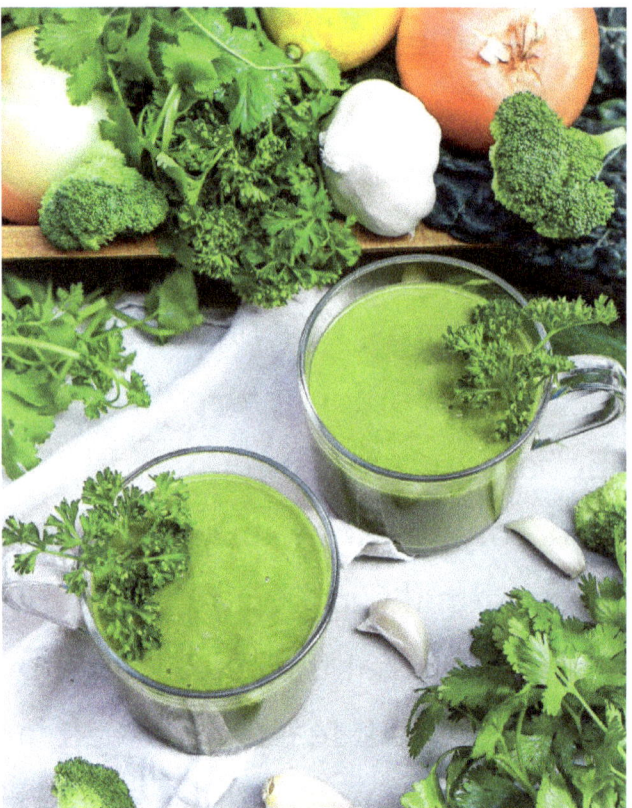

Ingredients

- Three medium or two large yellow onions,
- One zucchini
- Ten leaves dinosaur kale
- One head broccoli
- 4 cups vegetable broth
- One head garlic, cloves removed and minced
- ½ cup packed cilantro
- ½ cup packed parsley

- Juice of 1 lemon
- 3 tbsp raw, unrefined coconut oil
- 1/4 tsp sea salt

Process

In a pot, heat coconut oil over high until warm. Add onions and cook for 5-6 minutes, stirring occasionally, then add zucchini, broccoli, and kale and cook for 5-7 minutes more. Put the vegetable stock and bring to boil, then reduce heat to low and let it boil, covered, for 15-25 minutes or until broccoli is easily mashed with a fork. Put off the heat and then add garlic, and let cool, uncovered, for 15-20 minutes. Working in batches if necessary, blend with parsley, cilantro, sea salt, and lemon until very smooth.

38.   **Easy Garbanzo Beans Curry Soup**

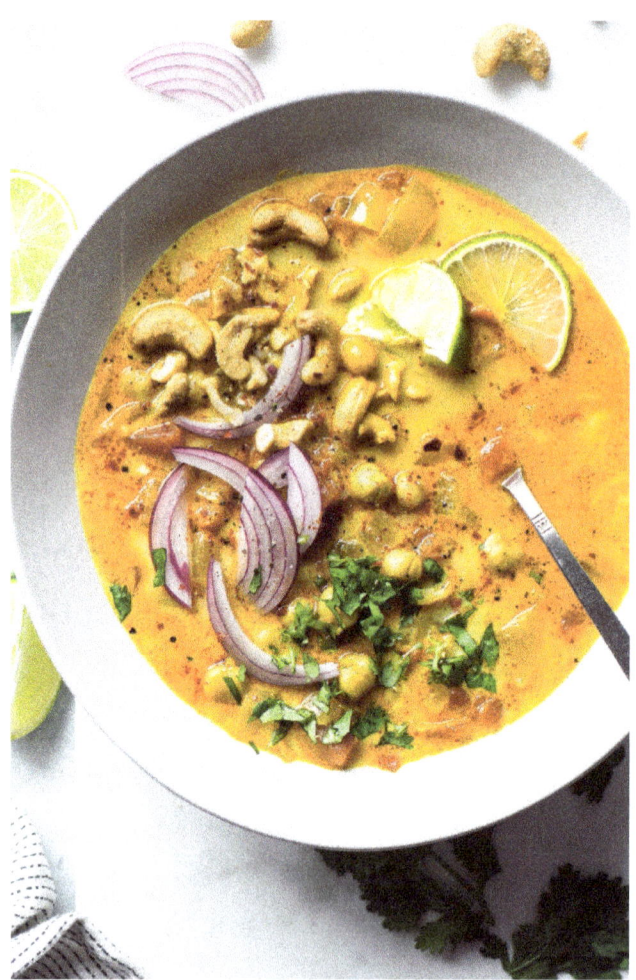

Ingredients:

- 1 cup canned garbanzo beans
- ½ cup chopped Swiss chard
- ½ large onion, chopped
- One medium tomato, chopped
- Two cloves of garlic

- ½ teaspoon turmeric powder
- ½ teaspoon coriander powder
- ½ teaspoon black pepper
- Two teaspoons olive oil
- ¼ teaspoon garam masala
- Salt to taste

Process

In a Pan, heat the oil and toss in the chopped garlic. Let it fry for 5-10 seconds, and then add in the chopped onions. When the onions turn goldish brown, add in the chopped tomatoes. Mash the tomatoes with the spatula. Add in turmeric, salt, black pepper, and coriander powder—Cook for a 1 or 2 minutes. Add in the can of garbanzo beans. Add one quarter cup of water, cover it with lid and let it cook for 5-10 minute. Remove the lid, add in the half cup of Swiss chard. Give it a stir, put the lid back up, and cook for 5-10 minute more. Remove from the heat. Sprinkle some garam masala on top, and your curry soup is ready!

39. Keto Broccoli Soup

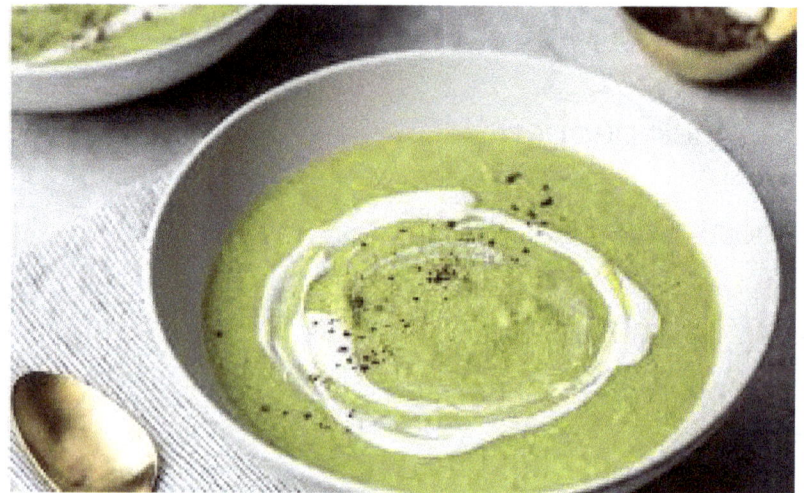

Ingredients

- 1 cup broccoli florets
- 2-3 cups of water
- ¼ cup fresh cream
- Two teaspoon butter
- ¼ cup chopped celery
- Two cloves of garlic, chopped.
- ½ teaspoon black pepper
- Salt to taste

Process:

Heat some butter in a pan. Put in some of the chopped garlic and cook until they turn goldish brown. Add in the celery and broccoli. Put and cook for 3-7 minutes over low-medium flame. Add pepper and salt. Put the vegetables in a blender and blend until you get a smooth paste. Put to a serving soup plate and add a generous amount of fresh cream.

40. Delish and Quick Thai Soup

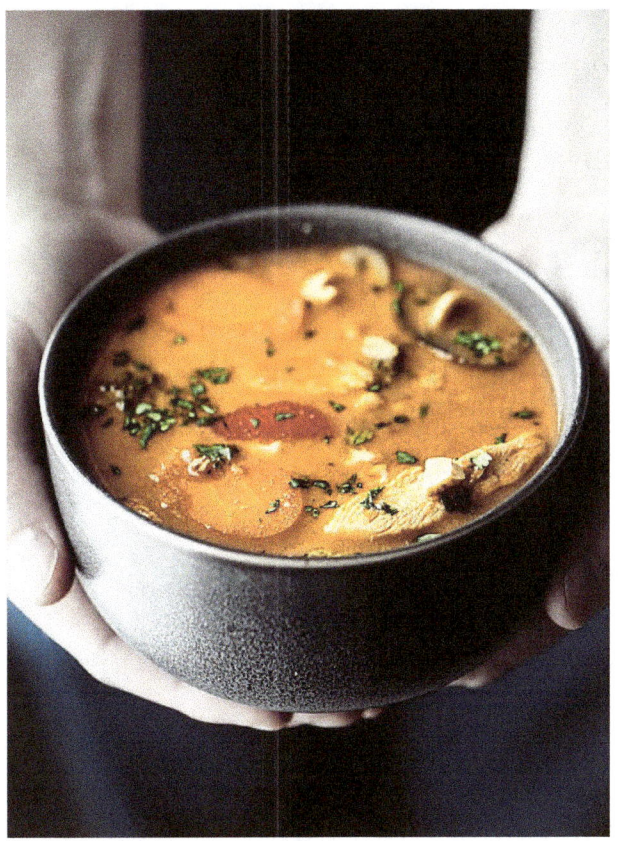

Ingredients:

- 1 cup cubed butternut squash
- ½ cup carrot, diced
- One medium-sized tomato, chopped.
- One medium-sized onion, chopped.
- 2 cups of vegetable broth

- 1-inch ginger, grated
- Two cloves of garlic, minced
- Two tablespoons Thai red curry
- ½ can of unsweetened coconut milk
- Juice of half a lime
- Two green chilies, sliced.
- One teaspoon brown sugar
- Two tbsp olive oil
- Salt as per taste

Process:

Add some olive oil in a pot over medium heat. Add in the minced garlic, chopped onion, and grated ginger—Cook for 2 minutes. Add in the butternut squash, carrots, and tomatoes—Cook for 2-5 minutes. Add the vegetable broth, lime juice, salt, Thai red curry paste, and coconut milk—cover and cook for 5-7 minutes. Put off the heat and stir in the sliced green chilies. Serve hot.

41. Italian Vegetable Soup

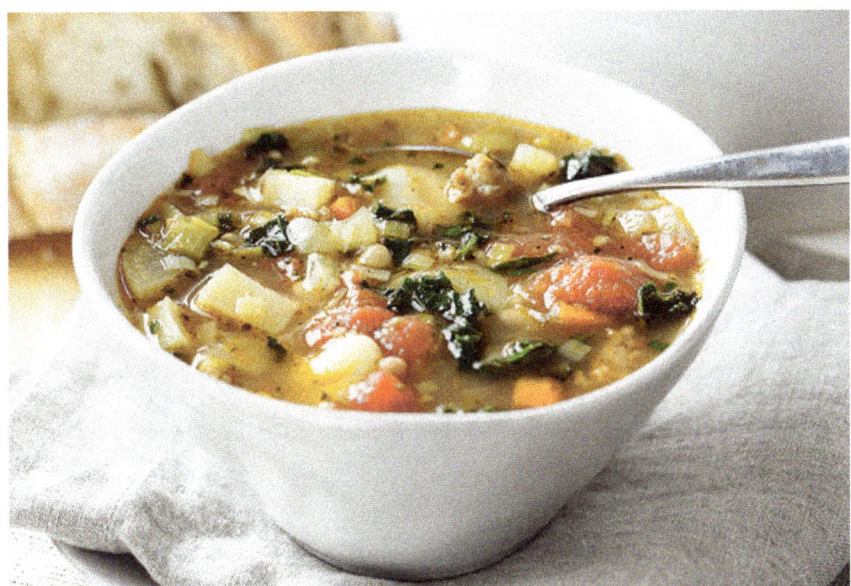

Ingredients

- ½ cup whole wheat pasta
- ½ cup chopped, ripe tomatoes
- One medium onion, chopped.
- ¼ cup carrot, chopped
- ½ cup celery, chopped
- One sprig of thyme
- One bay leaf
- 1 ½ cups vegetable broth
- Four garlic cloves, minced
- ½ cup canned butter beans

- Three tablespoons Parmesan, shredded
- One tbsp olive oil
- Salt as per taste
- ½ tsp Italian mixed herbs
- ½ tsp black pepper
- Fresh basil for garnish

Process

Add some olive oil in a pot over medium heat and add crushed garlic to enhance the flavor. Cook for 30-50 seconds and add chopped celery and onions. Cook for 2-5 minutes and add salt, tomatoes, carrot, and pepper. Stir in the vegetable broth. Put in some of the bay leaf and wheat pasta. Cover it with a lid and let it cook for ten minutes or until the pasta has been cooked. Open the lid, add some Italian mixed herbs, and give it a stir. Garnish with some fresh basil on top before serving.

42. Vegetarian Collard Greens Soup

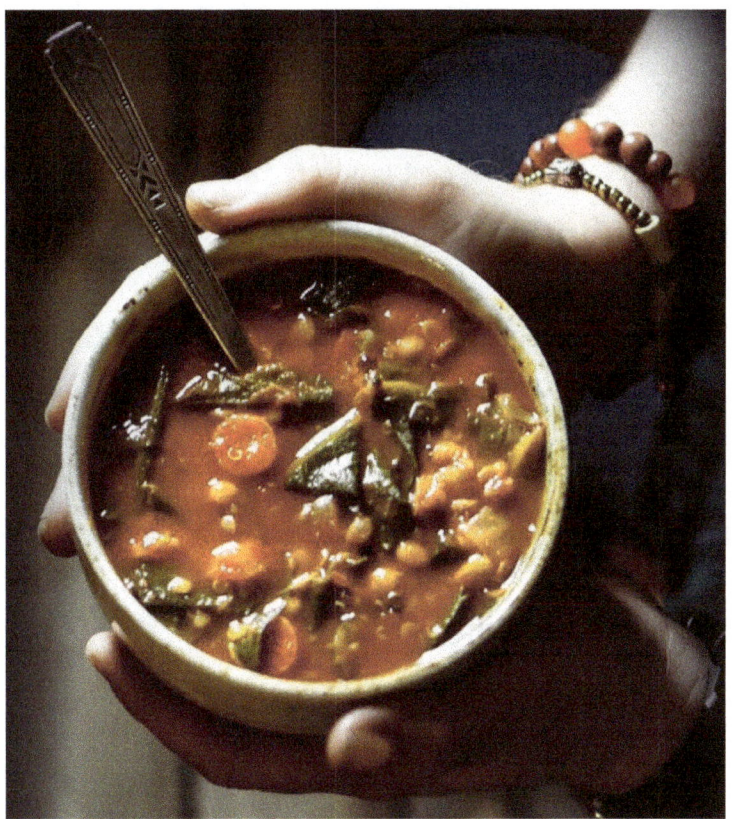

Ingredients

- 1 Tbs olive oil
- 2 tsp smoked paprika
- 1 tsp chili powder
- 1 tsp cumin
- pinch red pepper flakes
- One onion

- Three large carrots
- Three stalks celery
- 10 cups water
- 15 oz. Can no salt added diced tomatoes
- 6 oz. can no salt added tomato paste
- 2 Tbs lower sodium tamari or soy sauce
- 2 Tbs lemon juice
- 1 Tbs salt-free herb seasoning
- 1 Tbs sugar/sweetener
- One teaspoon roasted garlic granules or garlic powder
- 1/2 tsp salt
- fresh black pepper to taste
- 1 cup dried lentils
- 6 cups packed collard greens
- 1/4 cup uncooked quinoa

Process:

Prep the vegetables. Add oil into a large cooking pot. Add the cumin, red pepper flakes, paprika, and chili powder. Raise the heat to medium. Add the onion, carrots, and celery. Sauté for about 8-10 minutes. Add the water, and tomato paste, tamari or soy sauce, lemon juice, herb seasoning, sweetener, garlic granules, salt, pepper, and lentils. Stir to combine. Stir in the collard greens. Raise the heat to medium-high. Bring to a boil. Cover and turn the heat down to boil. Boil for 30 minutes, stirring occasionally. Stir in the quinoa. Simmer another 15-20 minutes.

Dinner:

43. Khichdi

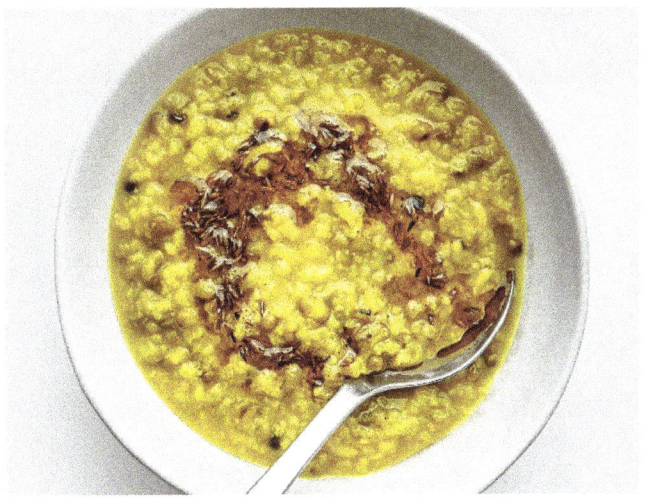

Ingredients:

- Half cup split green mung beans
- Half cup split pigeon peas
- Half cup any white long-grain rice
- One bay leaf
- One teaspoon of Black peppercorns
- One teaspoon ground turmeric
- One teaspoon Kosher salt
- ¼ cup unsalted butter

- Two teaspoons. cumin seeds
- Two dried red chiles
- Pinch of asafetida (optional, but good)
- Pinch of red chili powder

Process:

Combine Half cup mung beans and Half cup rice in a fine-mesh sieve and wash under cool running water until water runs clear. Transfer to a large pot and add one bay leaf, 1 tsp. Peppercorns, 1 tsp. Turmeric, 1 tsp. Salt, and 6 cups water. Boil over high flame, then reduce flames to medium-low and put a lid on the pot. Cook, scraping downsides, and giving the mixture a stir 15-20 minutes in, until rice and mung beans are tender and mixture just like a stew, 25-30 minutes. Turn off the heat taste and season it with salt if needed. Put it a side while you make the spiced ghee. For making the spiced ghee, melt a quarter cup of ghee in a pan over high flames. Add two teaspoons of cumin seeds and let them cook till seeds start to sputter and brown. Turn off the heat and immediately combine it with two dried red chiles, __ 1 pinch asafetida__ (if using), and one pinch red chili powder. Serve the kichri with some spiced ghee.

44. Bulgogi-Style Eggplant

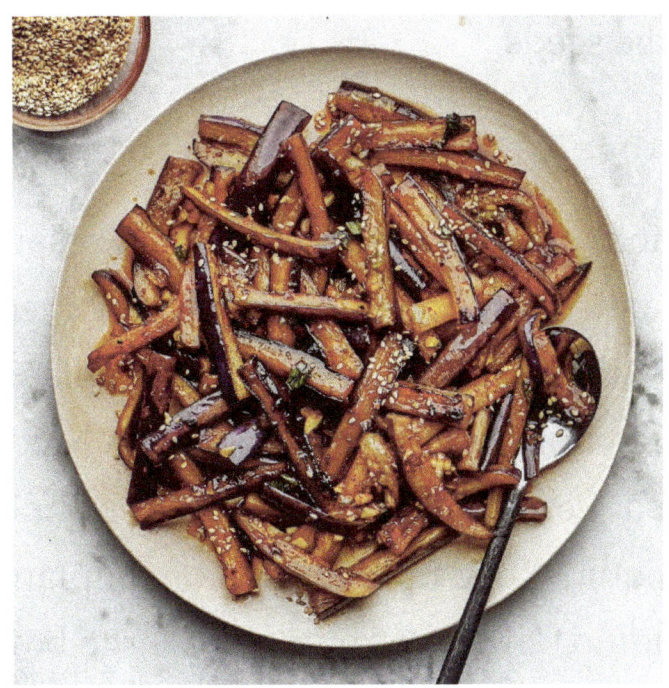

Ingredients:

¼ medium onion, finely chopped (about ⅓ cup)

Three garlic cloves, finely chopped

One scallion, chopped

¼ cup rice syrup, or 2 Tbsp. sugar

1 Tbsp. soy sauce

2 tsp. gochugaru (coarse Korean hot pepper flakes)

1 tsp. toasted sesame oil

1 Tbsp. Plus ½ tsp. kosher salt

1 lb. eggplants (preferably Korean)

1 Tbsp. vegetable oil

1 tsp. toasted sesame seeds

Process:

Mix rice syrup, onion, garlic, scallion, soy sauce, sesame oil, ½ tsp. Salt and gochugaru in a medium bowl until well combined. Cut eggplants crosswise into stips, then slice the pieces. Put eggplant strips in a medium bowl and combine 1 Tablespoon of Salt. Mix well by hand until all eggplant is salted. Let sit, mixing every 5 -20 minutes. Drain eggplant; discard liquid. Take up handfuls of eggplant, squeeze tightly to remove excess liquid, and then return to a large bowl. Add marinade to bowl with eggplant and combine well. Cover and chill for 25-30 minutes. Heat oil in a large, heavy pan over a medium-high flame and swirl to coat the pan evenly. Add marinated eggplant and spread evenly in the pan. Leave to set for a few minutes until the bottom is a little bit colored. Turn with tongs and cook until another side is lightly goldish, 3–5 minutes. Reduce flames to medium and continue to cook, pressing eggplant into pan and turning for regular intervals, until eggplant is cooked through and glazed. Any excess marinade has evaporated, 5–6 minutes — transfer eggplant to a plate. Sprinkle with sesame seeds. Serve hot or cold. Do Ahead: Eggplant can be made three days ahead. Store in an airtight container and chill.

45. Chinese Broccoli with Soy Paste

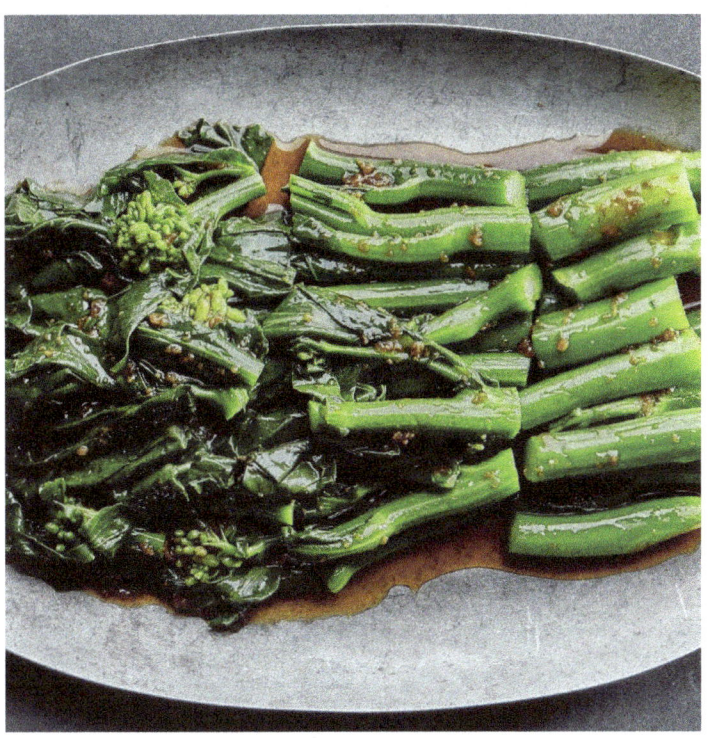

Ingredients

1 lb. Chinese broccoli

¼ cup soy paste

Process

Take a pot and place steamer basket in it and fill it with water, put on its lid, and let the water boil. Put broccoli into steamer basket, put on its lid, and steam broccoli until crispy, for about 5-10 minutes. Meanwhile, beat soy paste and 2 Tablespoon of water in a medium bowl. Arrange broccoli on a platter and drizzle sauce over.

46. Red Pepper, Potato, and Peanut Sabzi

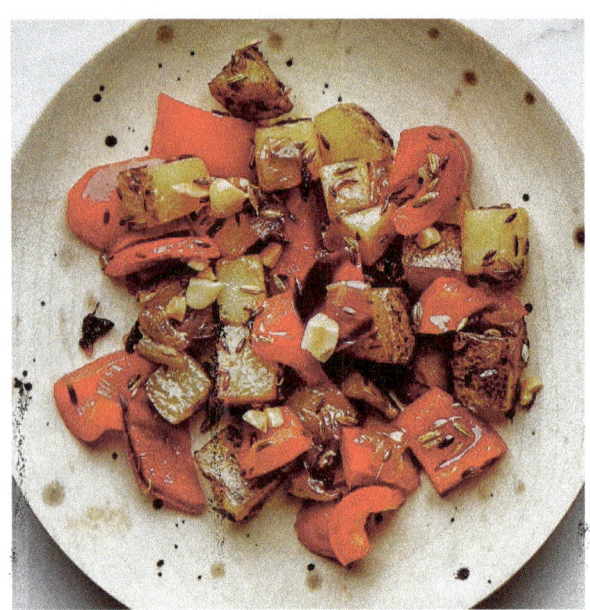

Ingredients

- 2 Tablespoon extra-virgin olive oil

- One teaspoon. cumin seeds

- One teaspoon. fennel seeds

- One small yellow onion

- One large russet potato

- Two medium red bell peppers

- One teaspoon. (or more) kosher salt

- ¼ cup roasted unsalted peanuts, crushed

- 1 Tablespoon fresh lime juice

Process:

Put some oil in a pan and heat it over a high flame until shimmer. Take some cumin seeds and let it cook for about 1-2mins until they turn a shade of brown. Reduce heat to medium flame and stir in fennel seeds. Add onion and cook, occasionally stirring, until translucent, 4–6 minutes. Put the potato and stir it, then spread the mixture evenly onto a pan. Cover and let it cook until potatoes are tender and not mushy for 5–10 minutes. Stir in salt and bell pepper. Put the lid at the pan and permit to heat till peppers are slightly softened 5–9 minutes. Using a spatula, scrape up the delicious charred bits from the pan's bottom and stir into the potato mixture. Put in peanuts and lime juice and stir the mixture. Taste and adjust lime juice and salt, if needed, before serving.

47. **Adobo-Style Eggplant**

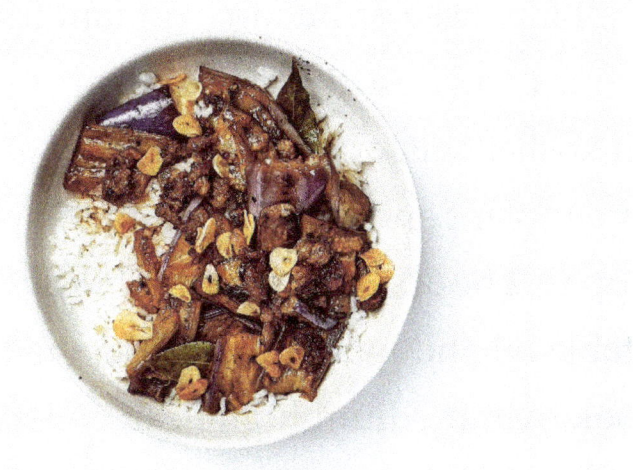

Ingredients

1 lb. small Japanese or Italian eggplant (about 3)

2 Tbsp. (or more) sugar, divided

One ¼ tsp. Diamond Crystal or ¾ tsp. Morton kosher salt, divided, plus more

One ½ tsp. freshly ground black pepper, divided

Eight garlic cloves

3 Tbsp. (or more) vegetable oil

4 oz. ground pork

3 Tbsp. coconut vinegar or unseasoned rice vinegar

2 Tbsp. soy sauce

Two bay leaves

Process:

Chop 1 lb. small Japanese or Italian eggplant into quarters lengthwise—place in a medium bowl. Add 1 Tbsp. Sugar, 1 tsp. Diamond Crystal or ½ tsp. Morton kosher salt, and ½ tsp. Freshly ground black pepper. Toss to evenly coat eggplant and let sit at room temperature for at least 20 minutes and up to 2 hours. Peel and thinly slice eight garlic cloves. Add 3 Tbsp. Vegetable oil and half of garlic to a medium Dutch oven or other heavy pot. Cook over medium-high heat, constantly stirring with a wooden spoon, until lightly golden and crisp, for about 5-10 minutes. Using a spoon, transfer garlic chips to a plate; season lightly with salt. Place 4 oz. Ground pork in the same pot and break up into small pieces with a wooden spoon. Season with ¼ tsp. Diamond Crystal or Morton kosher salt and cook, undisturbed, until deeply browned underneath, about 5 minutes. Using a slotted spoon, transfer to another plate, leaving the fat behind in the pot. Place eggplant on a clean kitchen towel and blot away any moisture the salt has drawn out. Working in batches Cook eggplant in the same pot until lightly browned adding more oil if needed, about 3 minutes per side. Transfer to plate with pork. Pour 1½ cups water into a pot and scrape up browned bits from the bottom with a wooden spoon. Add remaining garlic, 3 Tablespoon of Coconut vinegar, 2 Tablespoons of Soy sauce, two bay leaves, 1 tsp. Freshly ground black pepper and remaining 1 Tablespoon of Sugar. Bring to a simmer, then return pork and eggplant to the pot. Reduce heat to medium-low, partially cover, and simmer until eggplant is tender, silky, and sauce is reduced by half, 20–25 minutes. Season with pepper and salt and add a little more sugar if needed. Top with garlic chips and serve with cooked white rice.

48. Galayet Banadoura

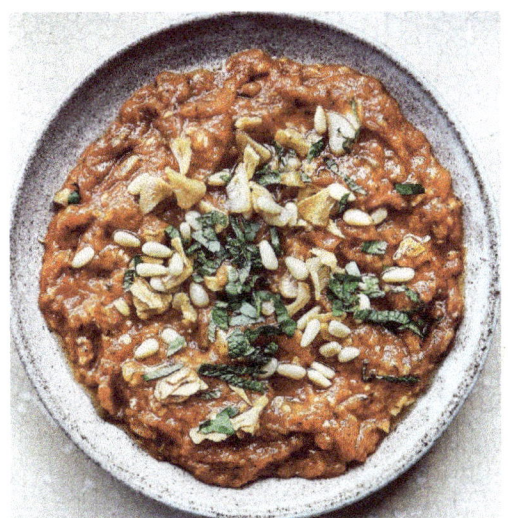

Ingredients:

800g plum tomatoes

Six tablespoon olive oil

One green chile, halved lengthwise, then roughly chopped, seeds and all

Eight garlic cloves: 2 crushed, six very thinly sliced lengthwise

Salt and black pepper

½ tsp dried mint

2 tbsp pine nuts

¼ cup/5g mint leaves, shredded

¼ cup/5g parsley leaves, roughly chopped

Process:

Take a Pan of water and bring it to a simmer over high heat, and put in the tomatoes. Cook for 3–5 minutes, then remove them with a spoon. While the tomatoes are still warm, peel off their skins. Once peeled, slice each tomato put them a aside. Put 3 tablespoons of oil into a medium pan and place over high heat. Add the tomatoes, chile, 1 tsp of salt, crushed garlic, and a good grind of black pepper. Cook for about 18 minutes, occasionally stirring, until the sauce has become thick. Put in some of the dried mint and transfer to a serving platter. Set aside to cool slightly.

Meanwhile, put the sliced garlic and the remaining 3 tbsp of oil into a small frying pan and place over medium heat — Cook until the garlic starts to become slightly golden. Put some of the pine nuts and cook for about 3-5 minutes. Put the mixture, along with the oil, over the tomatoes and garnish with the mint and parsley leaves. Serve warm or at room temperature. Keep the cooked tomatoes in the fridge for up to four days. The pine nuts and garlic can also be prepared well ahead and keep at room temperature. Present it on a dish.

49. Cauliflower Steaks

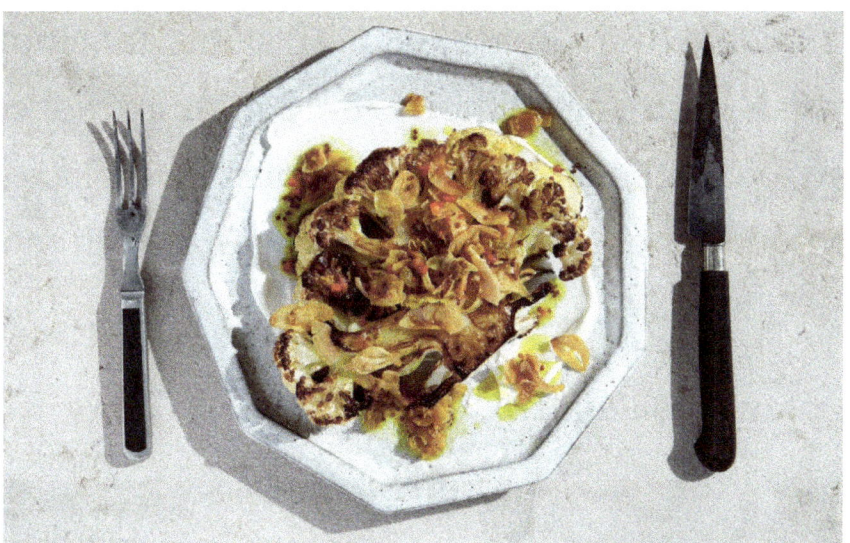

Ingredients:

- medium head of cauliflower
- 3 Tbsp. extra-virgin olive oil, divided
- Kosher salt, freshly ground pepper
- Plain whole-milk Greek yogurt and Coconut-Turmeric Relish (for serving; optional)

Process:

Preheat oven to 400°. Remove the toughest outer leaves from cauliflower (leave the tender inner leaves) and trim stem. Resting cauliflower on stem, cut in half from top to bottom, creating two lobes with stem attached. Trim off outer rounded edge of each piece to create two 1½"-thick steaks; reserve trimmed off florets for making cauliflower rice or roasted cauliflower. Heat 2 Tbsp. oil in a large cast-iron skillet over medium-high. Cook cauliflower, gently lifting up occasionally to let oil run underneath, until deep golden brown, about 5 minutes. Add remaining 1 Tbsp. oil to skillet, turn steaks over, and season with salt and pepper. Cook until second side is golden brown, about 3 minutes, then transfer skillet to oven. Roast just until stems are tender when pierced with a cake tester or toothpick, 8–12 minutes. Let cool slightly. If using relish, swipe some yogurt over each plate and place a steak on top. Spoon one-quarter of relish over each. Season with more salt and pepper.

50.   **Eggplant Lasagna**

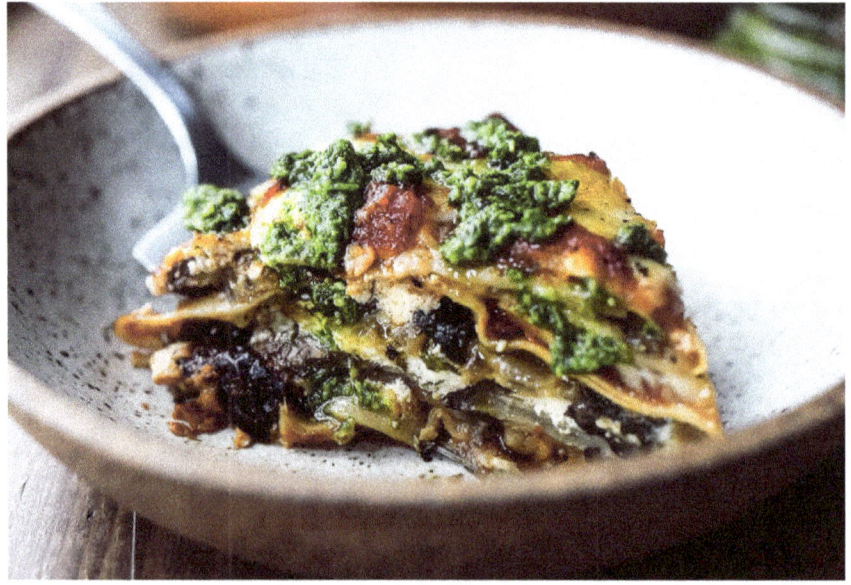

Ingredients

- 3 large eggplants (about 3 lbs)

- 1 teaspoon salt
- 2 tablespoons olive oil, spray olive oil or ghee
- 1 tablespoon olive oil
- one onion, diced
- 4–8 garlic cloves, rough chopped
- 6 ounces baby spinach, about 2 extra-large handfuls
- Salt and pepper to taste (1/4 teaspoon each)
- 16-ounce tub of whole milk ricotta (or sub tofu ricotta)
- 1 large egg
- 1/4 cup chopped basil
- 1/2 teaspoon salt
- 1/4 teaspoon nutmeg
- 1/4 teaspoon pepper
- 24-ounce jar marinara sauce, about 3 cups
- 8 no-boil lasagna noodles (or sub- gluten-free lasagna noodles)
- 1– 1 1/2 cups grated mozzarella (or meltable vegan cheese)
- 1/4– 1/3 cup pecorino (or parm, but I like pecorino better here)
- 1/4–1/2 teaspoon chili flakes (optional)
- 1 large garlic clove
- 1/4 cup toasted almonds, pinenuts or smoked almonds
- 1/2 cup packed basil leaves
- 1 cup packed arugula
- 1 teaspoon lemon zest
- 1 tablespoon fresh lemon juice
- 1/3–1/2 cup light flavored olive oil (make sure oil is not bitter)
- 1/4 teaspoon salt (if your almonds are heavily salted, use salt to taste.)

- 1/4 cracked pepper

Process:

Preheat oven to 400 F. Slice eggplant into 1/2-inch thick slices and place on two parchment-lined sheet pans. Sprinkle half the salt over the top as evenly as possible. Turn each piece over and sprinkle the remaining salt. Let the eggplant sit (and sweat) 15-20 minutes while the oven gets hot. When the eggplants look damp, pat the top side down with paper towels. Brush or spray with olive oil. Flip them. Blot with paper towels, spray with olive oil. Roast in the middle of the oven for 30-40 minutes, checking at 25 minutes. Roast until golden and tender. Thinner slices will cook faster, thicker slower. While the eggplant roasts, make the filling. In a large skillet, saute the onion, over medium heat until. tender about 5-7 minutes. Add the garlic and sauté until fragrant. Add the fresh spinach, lowering heat, gently wilting. Season with salt and pepper, turn heat off. In a medium bowl, whisk with a fork, the ricotta, egg, nutmeg, basil and salt. Set aside. Spray or brush a 9×13 baking dish (or 12-inch round baking dish) with olive oil. Place 3/4 cup marina sauce on the bottom, or enough to cover the bottom. Place the no-boil lasagna noodles over top. Spread another thin layer of marinara over the pasta, or just enough to lightly coat. Add half the roasted eggplant, overlapping a little if need be. Dot with half of the ricotta mixture. Spoon all of the wilted spinach mixture over top evenly. Sprinkle with 1/2- 3/4 cup mozzarella and 1/8 cup pecorino. Add another layer of pasta sheets. Lightly cover with 3/4 cup marinara (you'll need one more layer of marinara for the top, so if it looks like you could run out, water this down a bit here.) Next add the remaining eggplant, overlapping if need be. Smother with the remaining marinara sauce and spoon the remaining ricotta in fluffy dollops over the top. Sprinkle with a few chili flakes, 1/2 cup mozzarella cheese and 1/8 pecorino. Cover with foil (if your lasagna comes to the top edge of the baking dish, cover with parchment first and then with foil) and bake in a 375 F oven for 45-50 minutes, uncover and bake 10-20 more minutes, until golden and bubbling. While it is baking make the Arugula Pesto – place everything in food processor and pulse until combined, but not too smooth. Add more oil, to make it looser if you like, or less to make it thicker. The lasagna is done when it is golden, bubbling and slightly puffed in the center. Let it rest 5 minutes before serving, dot it with Arugula pesto or serve it on the side.

51.   nasi goreng

Ingredients:

- 8–12 ounces crispy tofu, pan-seared chicken or shrimp- all optional
- 3 tablespoons oil, divided
- 2 shallots (or 1/2 an onion), chopped
- 4 garlic cloves, rough chopped
- 1 cup diced carrot (small dice!)
- 1 cup red bell pepper, chopped
- 2 cups sliced mushrooms
- 1 cup fresh shucked peas, snow peas, snap peas or green beans

- 2 eggs, whisked with a generous pinch salt (optional)
- 3 cups cooked brown basimati rice, (leftover, dried out, see notes)
- 3 tablespoons soy sauce, more to taste (see notes) Or GF Liquid Aminos
- 1 1/2 tablespoons maple syrup, honey or palm sugar
- drizzle of sesame oil
- 1/4–1/2 cup chopped scallions

Process:

In an extra-large skillet or wok, pan-sear your choice of protein in oil with a little salt, pepper and chili flakes until golden and cooked through, set aside. In the same skillet, add 1-2 tablespoons oil and saute shallots, garlic, mushrooms, bell pepper and carrots over medium heat until the carrots are tender about 7-8 minutes. Season with salt. Toss in the fresh peas at the end. At the same time, while veggies are cooking, whisk, salt and scramble the eggs in a separate oiled pan, breaking the cooked apart into little pieces, set aside. (Or feel free to top with sunny side eggs after serving.) Once the veggies are tender, scoot them over to one side of the pan. Add a little more oil to the bare pan and add the rice. Turn the heat up and fry for 3-4 minutes, getting it a little crispy. Combine rice with the veggies. Drizzle with the soy sauce and maple syrup and mix well. Mix in the scrambled eggs and meat/shrimp/tofu if using. Taste and season with a drizzle of sesame oil, chili flakes, salt and pepper if needed. Stir in the scallions right before serving. Divide among bowls and serve with some of the optional garnishes, lime & chile paste.

52. indian shepherd's pie

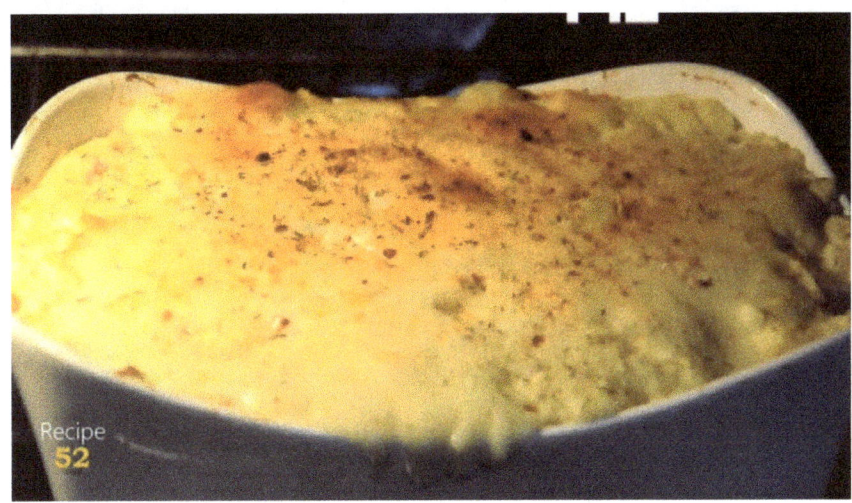

Ingredients:

- 2 1/2 lbs potatoes (Yukon gold, red, or any thin-skinned) (OR use 5 cups leftover mashed potatoes, with curry powder)

- 4 tablespoons, ghee, butter, vegan butter (ghee tastes the BEST)

- 1/2 cup plain yogurt (or sour cream)

- 1/2 cup milk, half and half or heavy cream

- 1 teaspoon salt, more to taste

- 1/2 teaspoon pepper

- 1-2 teaspoons yellow curry powder, more to taste

Filling

- 2 1/2 cups cooked lentils (3/4 cup -1 cup dry)

- 2 tablespoons ghee, or olive oil
- 1 large onion, diced
- 4 cloves garlic, rough chopped
- 2 cups diced carrot, (2-3 carrots)
- 2 cups diced celery (2-3 ribs)
- 2 teaspoons garam masala, more to taste
- 1 teaspoon cumin
- 1 teaspoon coriander
- 1 teaspoon salt
- 1/2 teaspoon pepper
- 2 teaspoons dried fenugreek leaves
- 1 cup veggie broth
- 1 cup frozen peas (or corn, or green beans- or use fresh)

Gravy:

- 2 tablespoon ghee or olive oil
- 1 teaspoon cumin seeds
- 1 teaspoon fennel seeds

- 3 tablespoons flour (or gf flour)
- 1 1/4 cups warm veggie broth

Process:

Cut potatoes in one-inch slices (if small, just in half) and place in a large pot. Cover with one-inch salted water. Bring to a boil, lower heat, cover and simmer until very tender about 20-25 minutes. Set lentils to cook in salted water (unless cooked already – and you could absolutely do this ahead) about 20-25 minutes (see notes) simmer until tender, but not falling apart, al dente. In a large 10-12 inch ovenproof skillet (or wide, shallow dutch oven) -heat the ghee over medium high heat and saute the onion 2-3 minutes, lower heat to med, add garlic, saute 2 mintues, add carrots, celery, cook 5-7 mintues. Add salt, cumin, coriander, fenugreek leaves and garam masala. Add broth. Bring to a simmer, cover and simmer on med low, until carrots are cooked through about 7-8 minutes. While this is simmering, MAKE THE GRAVY: Over medium heat, in a little pot, simmer the whole seeds (cumin seeds and fennel seeds) in ghee or oil until fragrant and golden. Add flour, whisking, stirring and toasting the flour one minute. Gradually whisk in the warm veggie broth. Cook until slightly thickened. Add this gravy to the filling, along with the peas and drained lentils. Mix to combine.

Taste the filling and adjust salt and pepper. Add more garam masala if you like. The filling should have thick stew-like, saucy consistency. If too dry, add a splash of broth or water. If too watery, simmer off some of that liquid. If the filling is too watery, the mashed potatoes will sink. Mash the potatoes: Drain the potatoes (saving some hot potato water) return to the same pot and mash with the 3-4 tablespoons ghee and yogurt. If potatoes seem dry or too stiff, add a little warm potato water to loosen. If you want extra richness a little milk, nut milk, half and half, or whipping cream is nice. I add about ½ cup. (Adding more yogurt will make these too tangy.) Season with salt, pepper and curry powder. Mash and whip until relatively smooth and light and fluffy. Taste and adjust salt. Place 8 big dollops over the lentils stew and fill in the spaces with smaller spoonfuls, carefully spreading out, maybe making a pattern with the back of the spoon, like frosting a cake. Place in the oven until golden and bubbling, about 20-25 minutes. Feel free to brown the top under a broiler. Garnish with scallions, chives or cilantro.

53. kimchi fried rice

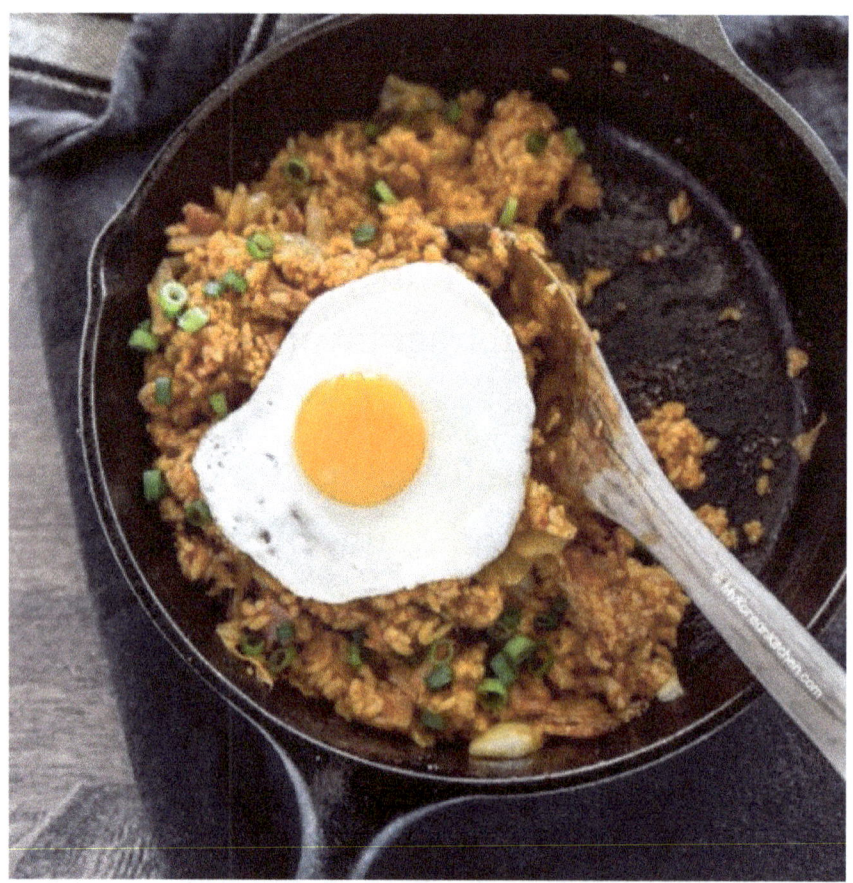

Ingredients

- 1–2 tablespoons oil (peanut oil gives this great flavor!)
- ½ cup onion- diced
- 2 teaspoons finely chopped ginger
- 1–2 cups chopped veggies – mushrooms, red bell pepper, zucchini, peas, carrots
- ½ cup kimchi– chopped, more to taste.
- 2 cups cooked, chilled rice
- ½ teaspoon soy sauce (optional, only if necessary)
- 1/2 teaspoon bonito granules (optional, but yummy!)
- salt and pepper to taste
- ¼ cup chopped scallions
- ⅛ cup cilantro
- 2 large eggs, poached, fried – or top with crispy tofu!
- Garnish with sriracha or hot sauce

Instructions

In a large skillet, heat the oil over medium-hight heat. Add onion and saute for 2-3 minutes, stirring, then turn heat down to medium. Add ginger and veggies. Saute until ginger is fragrant and veggies are tender, stirring often, about 5-7 minutes. Add chopped kimchi, and cook until heated through, about 1-2 minutes. Add rice, and continue cooking and stirring until warm and combined, about 3 more minutes.(Add a bit more oil or a little water if too dry.) Taste and adjust flavor by adding soy sauce, salt, bonito granules as desired. (*Kimchi adds a lot of saltiness, so add salt sparingly and to taste, as each kimchi is different. If tasting bland, add soy sauce.) Stir in the scallions. You could also stir in a handful of greens at this point, like baby spinach or arugula. Divide among two large bowls. Top with fried or poached egg. Sprinkle with cilantro and a generous squirt of Sriracha sauce. Serve immediately, breaking the yolk and letting act as a sauce over the rice.

54. aloo gobi (indian-spiced potatoes & cauliflower)

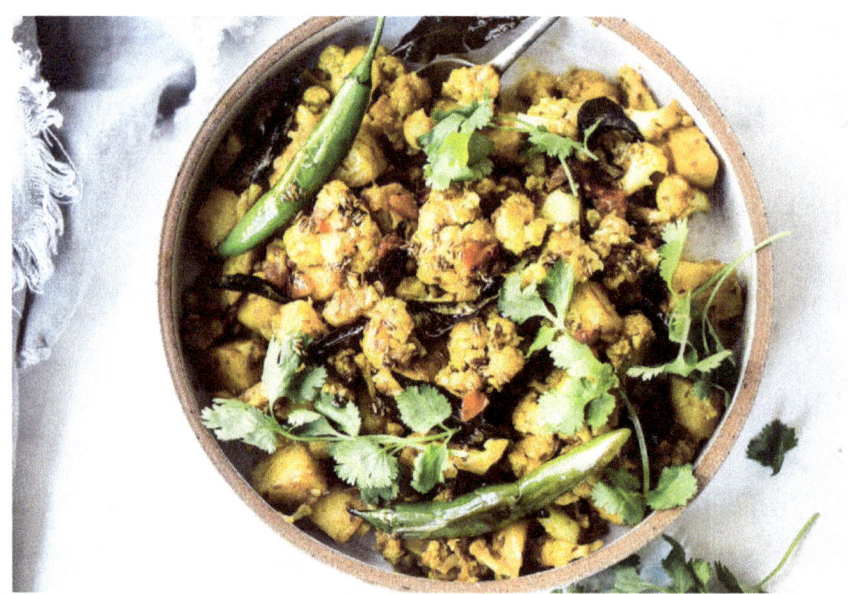

Ingredients

- 3 tablespoons ghee (or sub coconut oil or peanut oil– but ghee tastes best!)

- 1 shallot, chopped

- 4 cloves garlic, chopped
- 1 teaspoon fresh ginger, finely chopped
- 1 serrano chile, split down the middle, stem intact
- 8-10 curry leaves (optional)
- 2 teaspoon whole cumin seeds
- 1 teaspoon black mustard seeds
- 1/2 teaspoon ground turmeric
- 1/2 teaspoon paprika (or chili powder)
- 1/2 teaspoon asafoetida
- 1 teaspoons ground coriander
- 1 medium tomato, finely diced, with juices
- 3/4 cup water
- 1 teaspoon salt
- 2 cups diced potatoes (3/4 inch dice)
- 1 small head cauliflower, cut into small bite-sized florets (about 5 cups)
- Garnish: Cilantro or scallions

Instructions

Heat ghee in a large skillet over medium heat. Add shallot, garlic, ginger and serrano chili and saute until fragrant and golden, about 3-4 minutes. Add curry leaves, cumin seeds and mustard seeds and saute 1-2 minutes. Lower heat and add remaining spices – turmeric, paprika, asafoetida, coriander– along with tomato with its juices. Cook the tomatoes down on low heat for about 4-5 minutes until they begin to break down. Add salt and water, give a good stir scraping up any browned bits. Add potatoes and cauliflower, toss to coat. Cover, bring to a gentle simmer over med-low heat and cook, covered until fork-tender, about 15 minutes. Uncover and reduce, until all the remaining liquid is gone, stirring occasionally. You want this fairly dry (the ghee will keep it moist). Spoon into a serving dish, scraping all the goodness out of the bottom of the pan over top. Garnish with cilantro sprigs. Serve with naan, basmati rice or roti!

55. butternut lasagna with mushrooms and sage

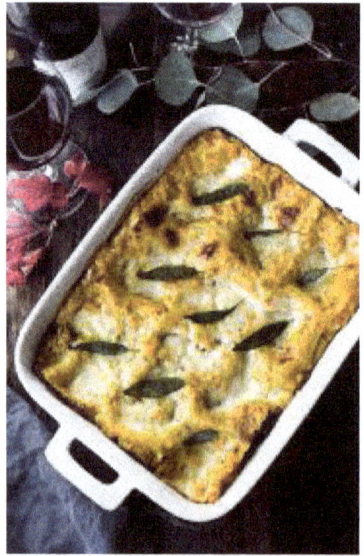

Ingredients

- Small butternut squash (2.5lbs – 3lbs) (you'll need about 4 cups, roasted)
- ½ a sweet onion, sliced into big wedges
- olive oil for drizzling

Mushroom Filling:

- 2 tablespoons olive oil or butter
- 1 ½ lb mushrooms, sliced (cremini, button, shiitake, portobello, wild mushrooms, etc.)
- 1 fat shallot or ½ onion, diced
- 4 garlic cloves, chopped
- 2 tablespoons fresh chopped sage
- ½ teaspoon salt
- optional – feel free to add a couple of handfuls baby spinach or greens and wilt them.

Ricotta Mixture:

- 1 lb ricotta cheese (or sub vegan tofu ricotta) If using the tofu ricotta, no need to add more salt or egg. Just nutmeg ☺
- one egg (optional)
- ½ teaspoon nutmeg
- ½ teaspoon salt

Butternut Puree:

- 3 tablespoons olive oil
- 3-6 tablespoons water
- 1 teaspoon salt
- ½ teaspoon pepper
- ½ teaspoon garlic powder
- 1 1/2 cups grated mozzarella cheese (about 3-4 ounces) or sub vegan "meltable" cheese
- ½ cup romano or parmesan (about 1 ounce) or sub vegan
- no-boil lasagna noodles (uncooked)
- Garnish with 9 crispy sage leaves (optional, see notes) or Arugula Pesto

Optional Quick Béchamel Sauce:

- 1 1/2 tablespoons olive oil (or butter)
- 1 ½ tablespoons flour
- 1 cup milk (or nut milk)
- generous pinch salt, pepper and nutmeg
- remaining ½ cup mozzarella and 2 tablespoons parmesan (or meltable vegan cheese)

Process:

Preheat oven to 425 F. Cut butternut squash in half, scoop out the seeds and place open side down on a parchment-lined baking sheet. Place sliced onion next to it and drizzle it with a little olive oil. Roast until fork-tender, about 30-40 minutes. Let cool. You could do this a day before or cook whole in an instant pot for 22 minutes. Lower oven to 375F In a large skillet, heat the oil or butter. Add mushrooms and shallots and salt, and saute over medium heat, until the mushrooms release their liquid and begin to brown. Add the garlic, sage and pepper. Cook until garlic is fragrant, about 2-3 more minutes, turn the heat off. You could toss in some spinach at the end and wilt for extra nutrients. Taste and make sure the filling has enough salt and pepper. You could also add a little truffle oil. You could make this 1-3 days ahead and refrigerate. Using a fork, mix the ricotta cheese with the egg, nutmeg and salt. (You really don't have to add the egg, but it adds a nice richness.) When the butternut is cool enough to handle, scoop all the flesh out into a food processor. You should have about 4 cups. Add the roasted onion, olive oil, water, salt, pepper and garlic powder. Puree until smooth. You will need at least 3 1/2 cups pureed and you want it to be almost *saucy*, like a marinara sauce (so add water if need be!). This will act as the "sauce". In a *greased* 9 x13 inch baking dish, add 1 cup of the butternut puree and spread out into a thin layer. Top with lasagna noodles. Add ½ of the ricotta mixture and spread out evenly. Top with half of the cook mushrooms. Sprinkle with ½ cup grated mozzarella and a couple tablespoons romano cheese. Add more lasagna noodles. Spread out the rest of the ricotta mixture as evenly as possible. Spoon half of the remaining butternut puree, erring on the side of less than half, so you have enough to cover the top (save at least 1 ¼ cups for the top.) Add the remaining mushrooms and all the good bits (onions and sage) and sprinkle with another ½ cup shredded mozzarella and couple tablespoons parmesan. Place the final noodles over the top. Lather with the remaining butternut puree and sprinkle with the rest of the cheese (or make the creamy béchamel sauce.- See notes.) You could assemble this 1-2 days before baking. Cover tightly with foil and **bake in 375 F oven for 40 minutes.** (If the foil touches the lasagna, place a layer of parchment between the foil and lasagna). Uncover and continue baking 15-20 minutes until golden and bubbly. Cut into 9 servings. Garnish with optional crispy sage leaves.

56.   Rigatoni with Easy Vodka Sauce

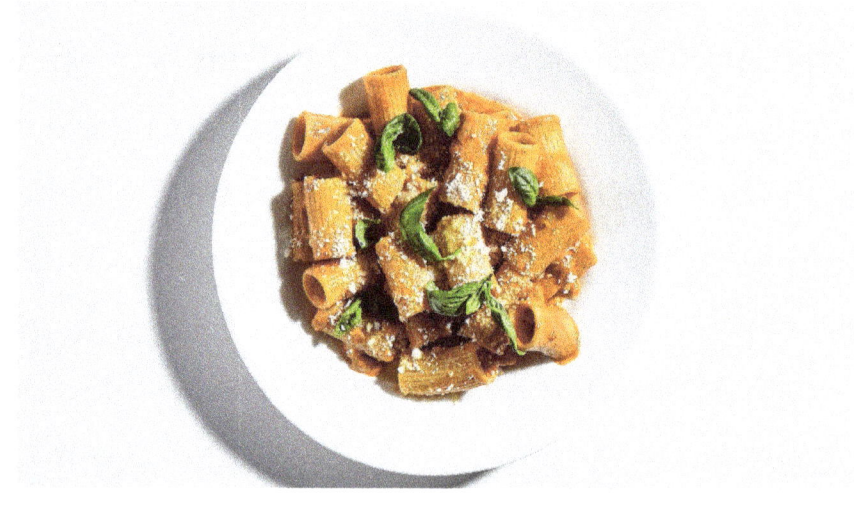

Ingredients

Kosher salt

1 medium onion

4 garlic cloves

4 oz. Parmesan cheese

2 Tbsp. extra-virgin olive oil, plus more for drizzling

14.5 -oz. tube double-concentrated tomato paste

½ tsp. crushed red pepper flakes

2 oz. vodka

¾ cup heavy cream

1 lb. rigatoni

Basil leaves (for serving)

Process:

Fill a Pot with 3-quarters of water and heat over high flames. Put in some **salt** and bring to a boil while you do your other prep. Peel and finely chop **one onion**. Firmly smash four garlic cloves with the flat side of a chef's knife and remove the peel. Shred **4 oz. Parmesan** on the smallest holes of the shredder. Heat **2 Tablespoons of Oil** in a Dutch oven over medium (position it next to a pot of water). Add onion and garlic and cook, continually stirring until onion starts to goldish-brown for 5–8 minutes. Add entire ½ **tsp. Red pepper flakes** and **4.5-oz. tomato paste** and stir until paste evenly coats onion.

Continue to cook, often stirring, until the paste is deep red and starting to brown on the bottom of the pot, 5-7 minutes. Add **2 oz—vodka** to deglaze the pan and stir to incorporate, scraping the pot's bottom. Reduce the heat to low. Scoop about quarter cup boiling water from the pot, then add **¾ cup heavy cream** to the measuring cup. Slowly add warmed cream to the Dutch oven, continually stirring, until a smooth sauce form. Remove from heat. Add **1 lb. rigatoni** to a pot of boiling salted water and cook accordingly to package instructions. About 1 minute before the timer goes off, use a heatproof measuring cup to scoop up about one cup pasta cooking liquid. Heat Dutch oven over low flame. Using a spider, transfer rigatoni to the Dutch oven along with any water that's on the pasta. Add half cup pasta cooking liquid to Dutch oven and stir to incorporate, then gradually add half of Parmesan, continually stirring to melt the cheese. Its best to use smooth, glossy sauce that coats each piece of pasta. Season with salt and add a splash of more pasta cooking liquid to thin sauce, if needed. Divide pasta among bowls. Top with the remaining cheese, spread evenly. Tear **basil leaves** over the pasta.

Desert;

57. Vegan Apple Cake

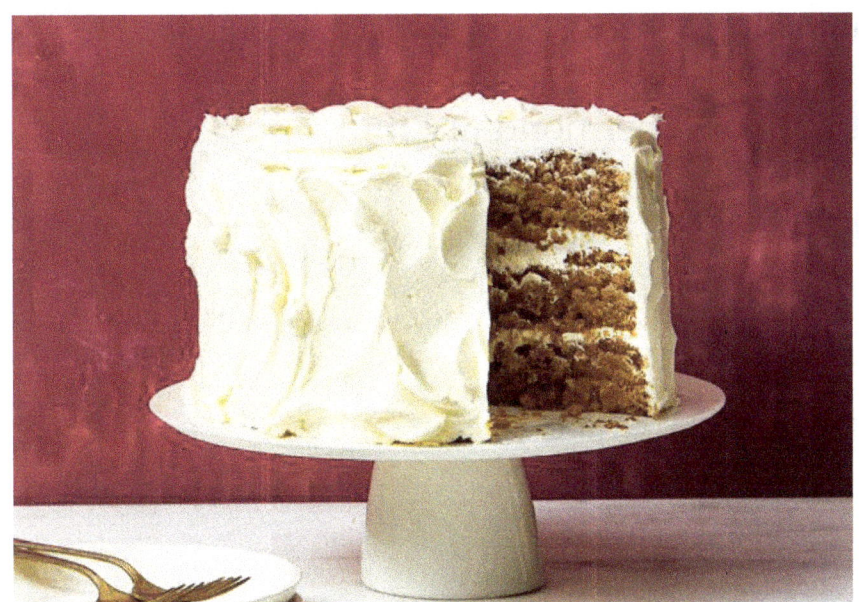

Ingredients

For cake

7 1/2 cup almond flour

1 1/2 cup potato starch

1/2 cup cornstarch

2 cup granulated sugar

3 tsp. ground cinnamon

2 1/4 tsp. baking powder

2 1/4 tsp. baking soda

1 1/2 tsp. ground allspice

1 1/2 tsp. ground ginger

3/4 tsp. ground nutmeg

1/2 tsp. kosher salt

2 1/2 cup oat milk or other nondairy milk

2 1/4 tsp. cider vinegar

3 tbsp. unsculptured molasses

1 1/2 tsp. pure vanilla extract

1/2 cup unsweetened applesauce

For frosting

3 cup apple cider

1 lb. vegan butter

1 lb. confectioners' sugar, sifted

Process:

Heat oven to 175 C. Lightly coats three 8-inch cake pans with non-stick cooking spray. Spray parchment on the bottoms with parchment. In a bowl, combine potato starch, almond flour, granulated sugar, cinnamon, baking powder, cornstarch, baking soda, allspice, nutmeg, ginger, and salt. In another bowl, mix vanilla, molasses, oat milk, and vinegar. Fold into the flour mixture and then fold in applesauce. Evenly divide about 2 1/3 cups batter among prepared pans, spread evenly, and bake until goldish brown and until a toothpick inserted into the center comes out clean, 25 to 35 minutes. Let the cake cool completely in pans. Meanwhile, prepare to frost:

In a small pan, boil apple cider until reduced to about two tablespoons for 25 to 45 minutes. Let cool. While cider syrup is cooling, remove vegan butter from the refrigerator and let it sit at room temperature for about 15-20 minutes but do not allow it to get too soft. If this happens, return to the refrigerator. By Using an electric mixer, beat reduced cider, sugar, confectioners' and vegan butter until fluffy and smooth, about 3-5 minutes. Makes about four and a half cups of frosting. (If it is too soft, return to the refrigerator to firm up.) Take a serving plate and put one cake layer put the bottom side up, and spread, heaping half cup frosting evenly over the top. Top with another cake, bottom side up; repeat. Spread remaining frosting over the cake evenly.

58. **Vegan Chocolate Chip Cookies**

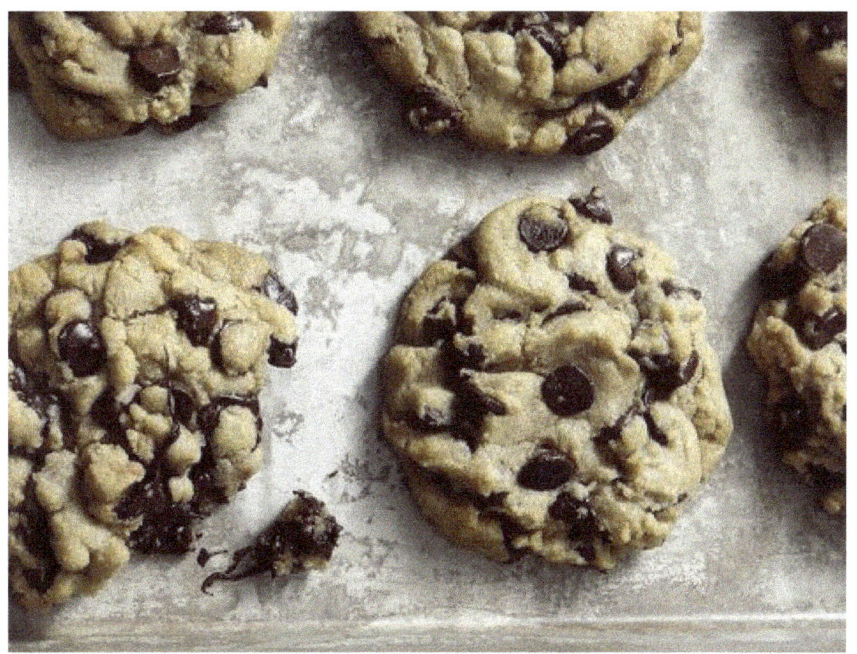

Ingredients:

2 cup all-purpose flour

1 tsp. baking soda

1/2 tsp. kosher salt

1/2 cup dark brown sugar

1/2 cup granulated sugar

1/2 cup canola oil

1/4 cup water

2 tsp. pure vanilla extract

1 cup bittersweet chocolate chips

1 cup semisweet chocolate chips

Process:

In a bowl, mix salt, baking soda, and flour. Toss with chocolate. In another bowl, break up brown sugar, making sure there are no lumps. Add granulated sugar, oil, water, and vanilla and whisk to combine. Add flour mixture and mix until just completely mixed (there should be no streaks of flour). Put two cookie sheets with parchment paper. Spoon out 2-inch mounds of dough, spacing 2 inches apart. Freeze 30 minutes. Heat oven to 375°F. Bake cookies, rotating position of pans after 6 minutes until edges are golden brown, 9 to 12 minutes total. Let cool.

59. VEGAN ALMOND JOY BAR

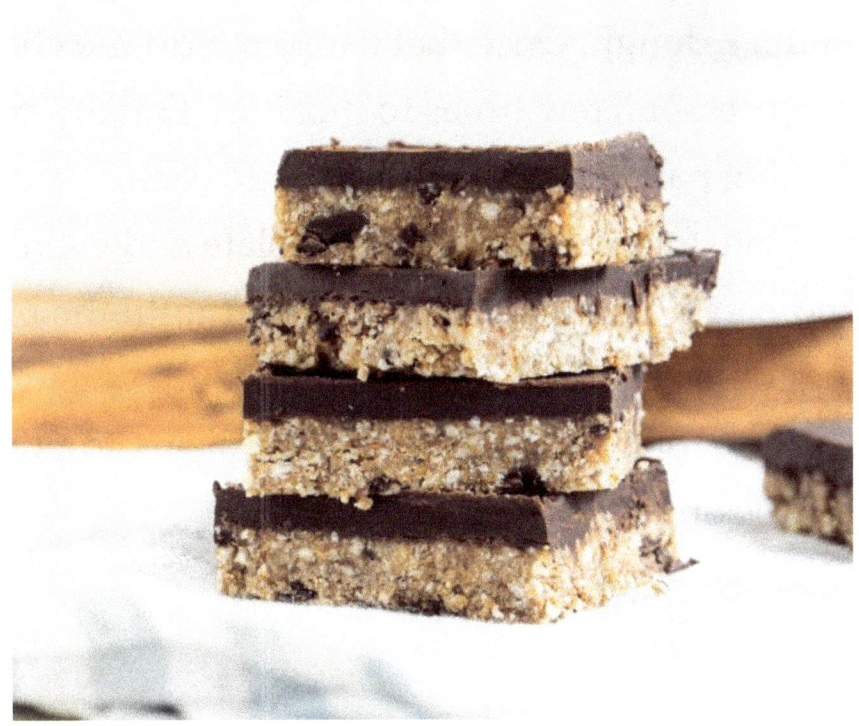

Ingredients

- Coconut.
- Chocolate.
- Almonds.
- Dates.

Directions:

Put the shredded coconut to your food processor and blend for 7-10 minutes until it forms a paste. It doesn't need to be as slushy as coconut butter, but it should resemble a thick, grainy paste. Add the almonds and dates to the food processor with the coconut paste and combine until it forms a thick dough. Once that's mixed, add the chocolate and pulse the food processor a few times to mix it in. Equally press the dough into a baking pan, firmly pressing it into each corner. If you're adding the chocolate topping, melt the chocolate and evenly spread it over the almond bars. Put the pan in the freezer until the bars are firm. If you are going to add chocolate on top, make sure you let the bars sit at room temperature for 15-25 minutes before slicing to prevent the chocolate from cracking when you cut it.

60. **No-Bake Vanilla Cake Bites**

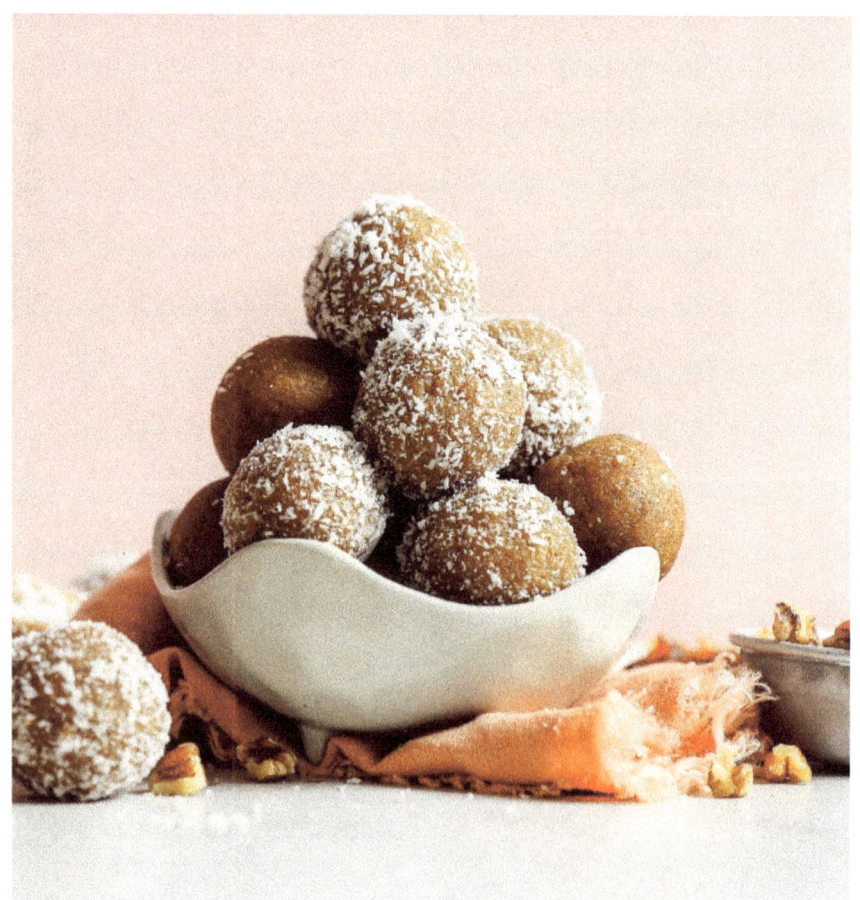

Ingredients:

- 1 1/4 cups Medjool dates
- 1 1/4 cups raw walnuts
- 1 cup almond flour
- 1/3 cup coconut flour
- Pinch sea salt
- Two teaspoon vanilla extract
- Finely shredded unsweetened coconut *(optional)*

Process

Pulse pitted dates in a food processor until small bits remain. Take it out from the food processor and placed it apart. Add the almond flour, walnuts, coconut flour, and sea salt into the food processor. Blend till a semi-high-quality meal is carried out. Add dates returned in addition to the vanilla extract. Pulse until loose dough form. Be careful not to over-blend. You're looking for pliable dough, not a purée. Using a cookie scooper, scoop out 2-Tablespoon amounts and roll into balls with hands or release lever on the scoop and place directly on a parchment-lined baking sheet. Repeat until all dough is used up. Roll in finely shredded coconut, or leave it as is. Store in refrigerator or freezer. Keep in the fridge for up to 6-7 days or in the freezer for up to 3-4 weeks. You can also make a loaf from the dough or 6×6-inch cake pan and slice it into bars.

61. **Chilled Chocolate Torte**

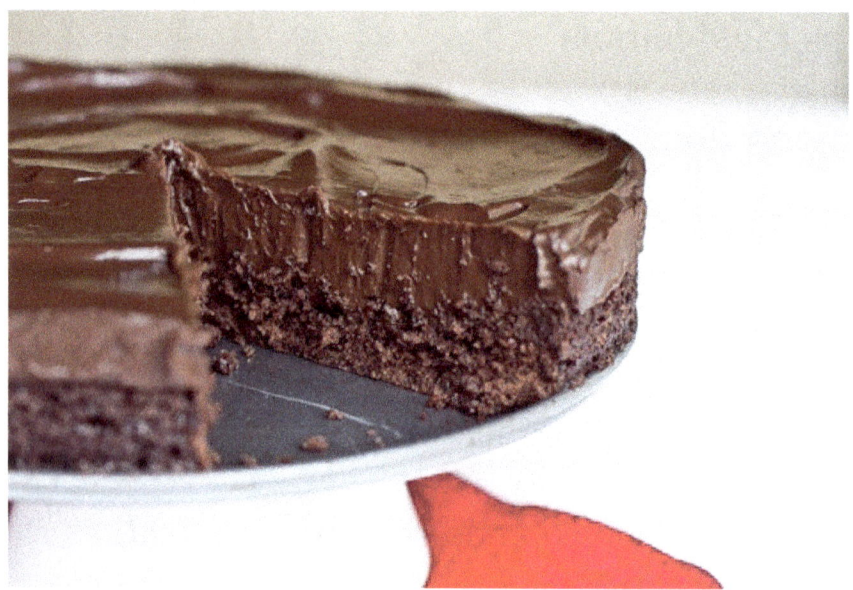

Ingredients:

Toasted Hazelnut Crust

- 3/4 cup raw hazelnuts
- 1/4 cup coconut oil
- 3 tablespoons maple syrup
- 1/4 teaspoon fine-grain sea salt
- 1/2 cup gluten-free oat flour
- 1/2 cup gluten-free rolled oats

Chocolate Filling

- 1 1/2 cup cashews
- 3/4 cup pure maple syrup

- 1/2 cup coconut oil
- 1/3 cup cocoa powder
- 1/3 cup dark chocolate chips, melted
- 2 teaspoons pure vanilla extract
- 1/2 teaspoon fine-grain sea salt
- 1/2 teaspoon espresso powder

Toppings (optional)

- Shaved chocolate
- Coconut flakes

Process

Make the Toasted Hazelnut Crust

Preheat the oven to 170- 175 C. Lightly grease a nine-inch pie dish with coconut oil. In a food processor, put the hazelnuts right into a high-quality crumb with the texture of sand. Add the oil, maple syrup, salt, and oat flour and process once more until the dough comes together. Add the oats and pulse them until the oats are chopped but nevertheless have a few textures to them. The dough has to stick collectively slightly while pressed between your fingers, but it shouldn't be super-sticky. If it's too dry, add 1 teaspoon water or processing a bit longer. With your fingers, mesh apart the dough evenly over the bottom of the pie dish. Starting from the center, press the mixture firmly and evenly into the dish, transferring outward and upward alongside the side of the pie dish. The harder you press the crumbs into the dish, the better the crust will hold together. Poke some fork holes into the bottom to allow steam to get out. Bake the crust, exposed, for 10 to 15 mins, until lightly golden. Removed from the oven and set apart to chill on a rack for 15 to 25 minutes.

To make the filling

Wash the cashews. In a blender, mix the espresso powder, cocoa powder, melted chocolate, agave, oil, vanilla, salt, and soaked cashews and blend it until the filling is completely smooth. It can take 1-3 minutes of blending to get it smooth. Add a tbsp of almond milk to help it along if the blender needs more liquid to get it going. Put the filling into the prepared crust, taking every last bit out of the blender. Smooth out the top evenly. Garnish with chocolate and/or coconut flakes, if desired. Place a dish on a even surface in the freezer, uncovered. Freeze for a 2-3 hours, and then cover the dish with foil and freeze for 4-8 more hours until the pie sets. Take out the pie from the freezer and put it on the counter for 5-10 minutes before slicing. This pie is should be served frozen. Wrap left over slices individually in foil and store them in an airtight container in the freezer for 1 week.

62. Peanut Butter Protein Balls

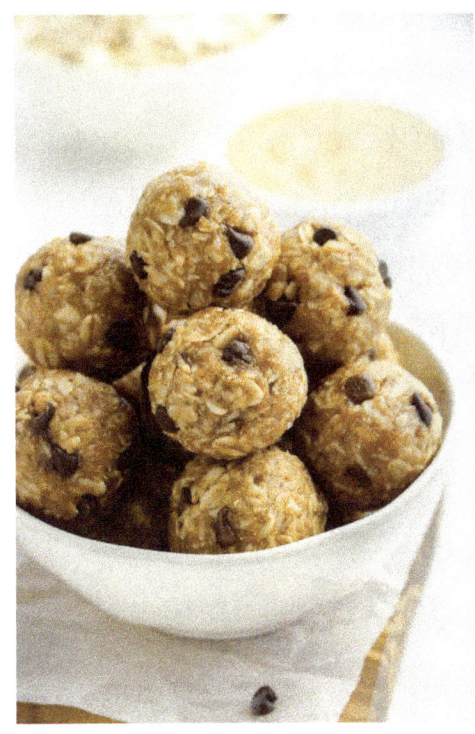

Ingredients

- 1 cup large Medjool dates pitted
- 2-4 tablespoons water
- 1 cup peanut flour
- 3/4 cup oats
- 1/2 cup roasted peanuts
- 1/4 cup natural peanut butter
- 2 tablespoons flax seeds ground into meal
- pinch of salt

- 1/4 cup chocolate chips optional

Process:

Put the pitted dates in about 2 cups of water for 25- 30 minutes. Drain, reserving the water. In a food processor combination dates with 2-four tablespoons of water, slowly adding water as wanted and scraping down the edges frequently till a paste has formed. Add peanut butter, peanuts, salt, flax seeds, peanut flour, and oats and blend together into a thick dough. Round out about 2 tbsp of dough into balls and place on a parchment-lined baking sheet. Refrigerate for 1 hour until firm. Store in an airtight container in refrigerator up to 5 days or in the freezer for 1 month.

63. **Cinnamon Walnut Apple Cake Baked with Olive Oil**

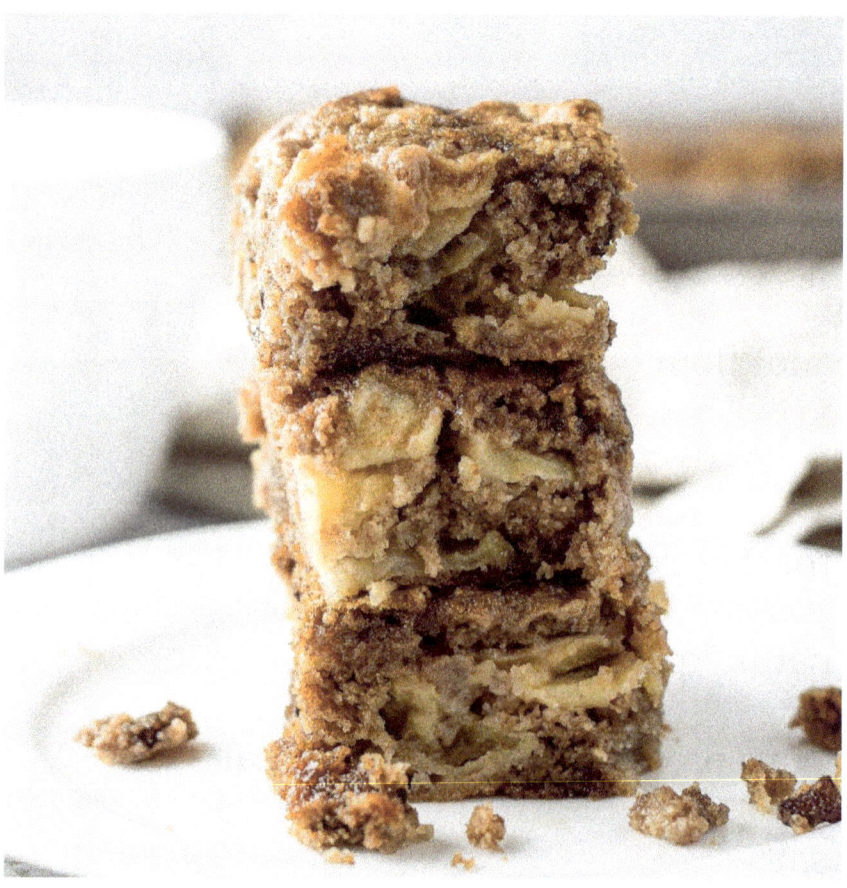

Ingredients

- 4 eggs
- 1 cup earthy colored sugar (in addition to 2 Tablespoons for apples)
- 1 cup additional virgin olive oil
- 1 cup milk
- 2 1/2 cups wheat flour
- 2 teaspoons preparing powder
- 1 teaspoon vanilla concentrate
- 4 apples, stripped, split, cored, and daintily cut
- 1/2 cup pecans, cleaved
- 1/2 cup raisins
- 1/2 teaspoons ground cinnamon
- 3 tablespoons sesame seeds

Instructions

Preheat stove to 375 degrees. Beat eggs and sugar with a hand blender for 10 minutes. Add olive oil and beat for an extra 3 minutes. Add milk, wheat flour, preparing powder and vanilla. Beat for 2 minutes. Brush a 9" cake container with olive oil. Add a large portion of the hitter to the skillet. In a bowl, blend apples, 2 tablespoons of earthy colored sugar, pecans, raisins and cinnamon. Pour apple combination on top of hitter in cake skillet. Add remaining hitter to container and sprinkle with sesame seeds. Heat for 45-50 minutes until embedded blade confesses all.

64. GREEK YOGURT CHOCOLATE MOUSSE

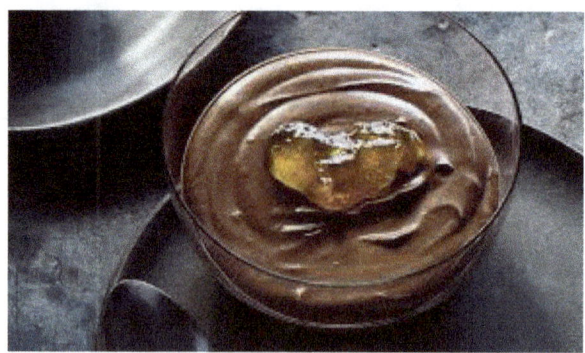

INGREDIENTS

- 180ml/3/4 cup milk
- 100g/3 1/2 oz dull chocolate
- 500ml/2 cups greek yogurt
- 1 tbsp nectar or maple syrup
- 1/2 tsp vanilla concentrate

Process:

Empty the milk into a pot and add the chocolate, either ground or finely cleaved or shaved. Tenderly warmth the milk until the chocolate softens, being mindful so as not to allow it to boil. When the chocolate and milk have completely joined, add the nectar and vanilla concentrate and blend well. Spoon the greek yogurt into a huge bowl and pour the chocolate blend on top. Combine as one well prior to moving to singular dishes, ramekins or glasses. Chill in the ice chest for 2 hours. Present with a little spoonful of greek yogurt and some new raspberries. The chocolate mousse will keep in the cooler for 2 days.

65. Fig and pistachio cake

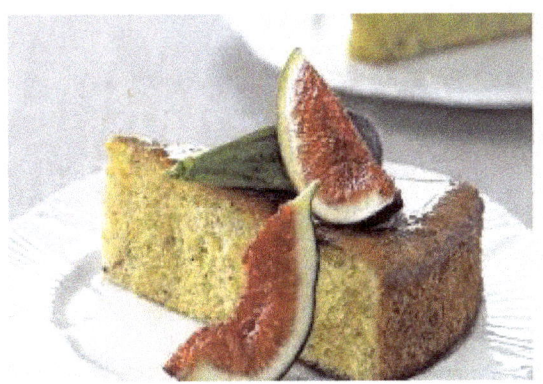

Ingredients

For pistachio cake

- 40 g pistachios
- 75 g powdered sugar
- 40 g blanched almonds
- 40 g egg yolks
- 60 g eggs
- 115 g egg whites
- 2 g cream of tartar
- 50 g + 1/2 cup sugar
- 60 g all-purpose flour

For mascarpone frosting

- 1 cup heavy cream
- 8 oz. mascarpone cheese
- 1/2 cup powdered sugar

For roasted figs

- About 12 ripe figs
- 1 tablespoon unsalted butter
- 2 tablespoons honey

Instructions

For the cake:

Preheat oven to 425 degrees F. Grease two 8x8 pans, line with parchment paper, and grease parchment paper. Combine pistachios, powdered sugar, and almonds in a food processor. Process until nuts are finely ground. Pour nut mixture into a large mixing bowl. Add in eggs and egg yolks and stir until combined. Combine egg whites, cream of tartar, and 2 tablespoons of the 50 g of sugar in bowl of a stand mixer. Whip until soft peaks form. Add remaining sugar and whisk until stiff peaks. Sift the flour over the nut mixture and stir to combine. Add in the egg whites and carefully fold in. Divide the batter between the two pans. Bake for 8-10 minutes until the tops are lightly colored and the top just springs back to the touch. Remove from oven and place on wire racks. Run an offset spatula or knife around the edges to loosen the cake from the pans. Let cool. For the sugar syrup: Combine the remaining 1/2 cup sugar and 1/2 cup water in a medium saucepan on the stove and bring to a boil, stirring to let the sugar dissolve. Let cool.

For mascarpone frosting:

Combine all ingredients in bowl of a stand mixer. Whisk together until soft peaks form. Add more confectioner's sugar if you would like it sweeter. Do not over whisk or the mixture will curdle. To assemble the cake: Trim off the edges of each square of edge to even them off. Place one layer of cake on a plate. Brush a little of sugar syrup over the cake layer. Spread a layer of frosting evenly on top. Place second layer of cake on frosting and brush sugar syrup over it. Spread a layer of frosting evenly on top. Refrigerate cake for about an hour or so to let frosting set. When you are ready to serve the cake, you can take it out and trim the sides so they look nice and even.

For the figs:

Preheat oven to 425 degrees F. Wash figs and slice them in half. Arrange in an ovenproof baking dish just large enough to fit them. Combine butter and honey in a small saucepan and cook over medium heat on the stove until butter is melted. Pour over the figs. Place figs in oven and bake for about 13-15 minutes, until the sauce is bubbling. Remove figs and let cool on wire rack for a few minutes before serving.

66. Sticky Gluten-Free Lemon Cake

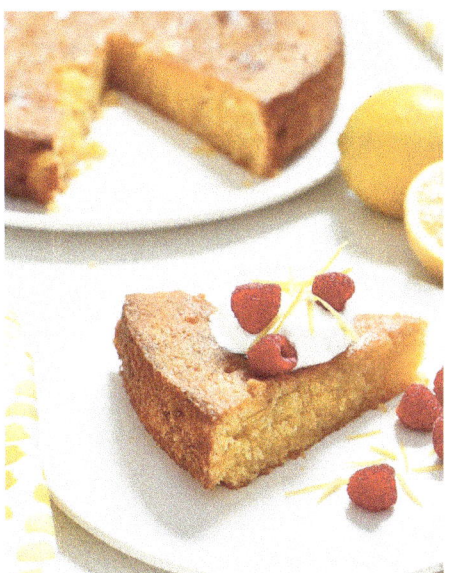

INGREDIENTS

For the cake:

- 2 cups almond flour
- 3/4 cup polenta
- 1/2 teaspoons heating powder
- 1/4 teaspoon salt
- 14 tablespoons (7 ounces) unsalted margarine, at room temperature, in addition to additional for the skillet
- 1 cup granulated sugar
- 3 enormous eggs
- Finely ground zing of 2 medium lemons
- 1/2 teaspoon vanilla concentrate

For the syrup and serving:

- 1/2 cup powdered sugar
- 3 tablespoons newly crushed lemon juice
- Whipped cream, for serving (discretionary)

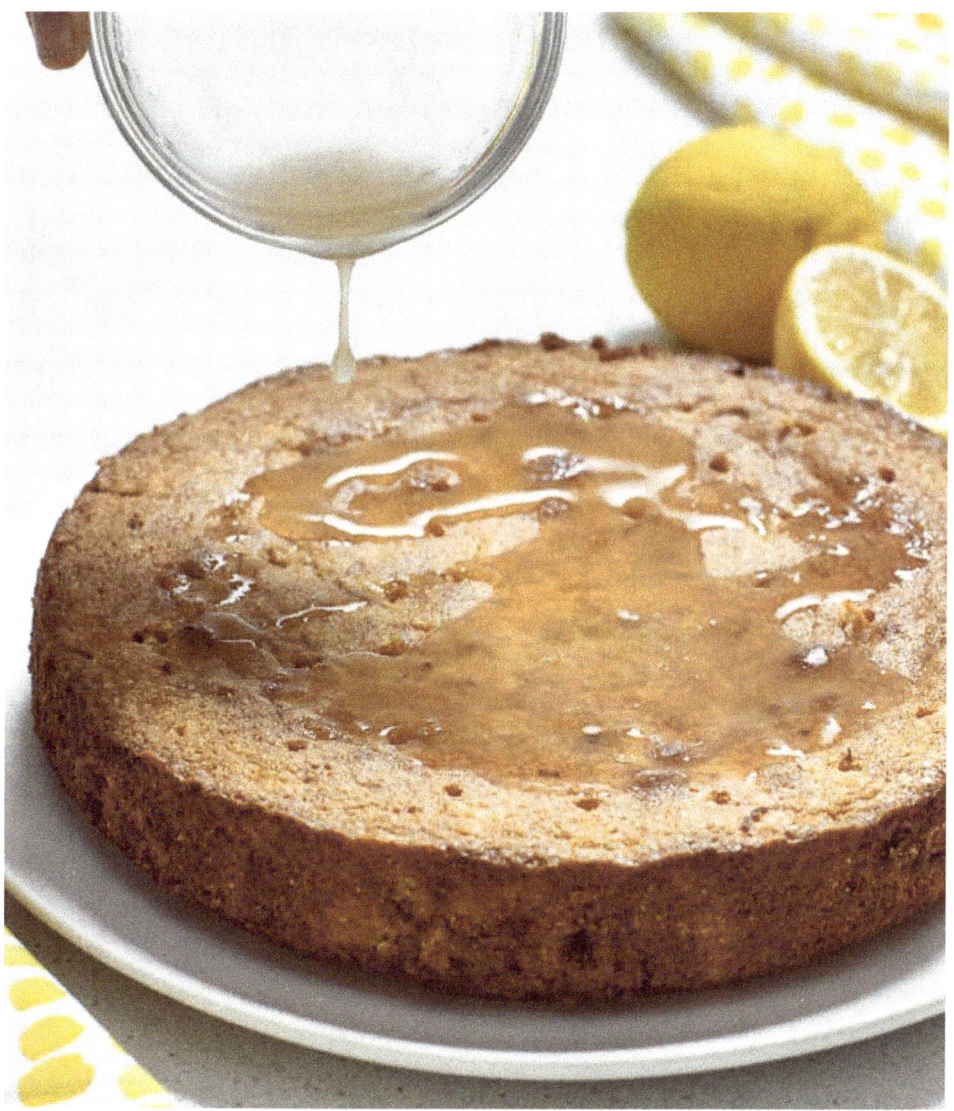

Process:

For cake:

Organize a rack in the stove and warmth to 350°F. Line the lower part of a 9-inch spring form skillet with material paper. Coat the paper and sides of the container with margarine; put in a safe spot. Spot the almond flour, polenta, heating powder, and salt in a medium bowl and race to consolidate; put in a safe spot. Spot the margarine and sugar in the bowl of a stand blender fitted with the oar connection. (Then again, utilize an electric hand blender and huge bowl.) Beat on medium speed until helped in shading, around 3 minutes. With the blender on medium speed, add 1/3 of the almond flour combination and beat until fused. Beat in 1 egg until consolidated. Keep beating in and substituting the leftover almond flour blend and eggs in 2 additional options. Stop the blender and scratch down the sides of the bowl with an elastic spatula. Add the lemon zing and vanilla concentrate and beat until just consolidated. Move the hitter to the container and spread into an even layer. Heat until the edges of the cake has started to pull away from the sides of the skillet, around 40 minutes. Spot the skillet on a wire rack and make the syrup.

For the syrup:

Spot the powdered sugar and lemon juice in a little pot over low warmth and cook, mixing periodically, until the powdered sugar is totally broken up and the syrup is warm. Eliminate from the warmth. Utilizing a toothpick, punch holes everywhere on the cake, dispersing the openings around 1-inch separated. Gradually shower the warm syrup uniformly over the cake. Allow the cake to cool totally, around 1/2 hours. Eliminate the sides of the skillet, cut into wedges, and present with whipped cream whenever wanted.

67. Balsamic Berries with Honey Yogurt

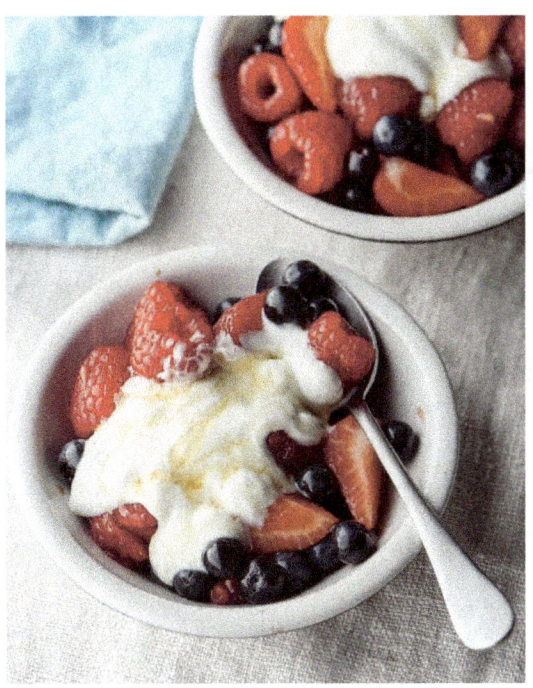

INGREDIENTS

- 8 ounces strawberries, hulled and split, or quartered if extremely enormous (around 1/2 cups)
- 1 cup blueberries
- 1 cup raspberries
- 1 tablespoon balsamic vinegar
- 2/3 cup entire milk plain Greek yogurt
- 2 teaspoons nectar

Process:

Throw the strawberries, blueberries, and raspberries with the balsamic vinegar in a huge bowl. Let it sit for 10 minutes. Mix the yogurt and nectar together in a little bowl. Split the berries between serving bowls or glasses and top each with a spot of nectar yogurt.

68. Blood Orange Olive Oil Cake

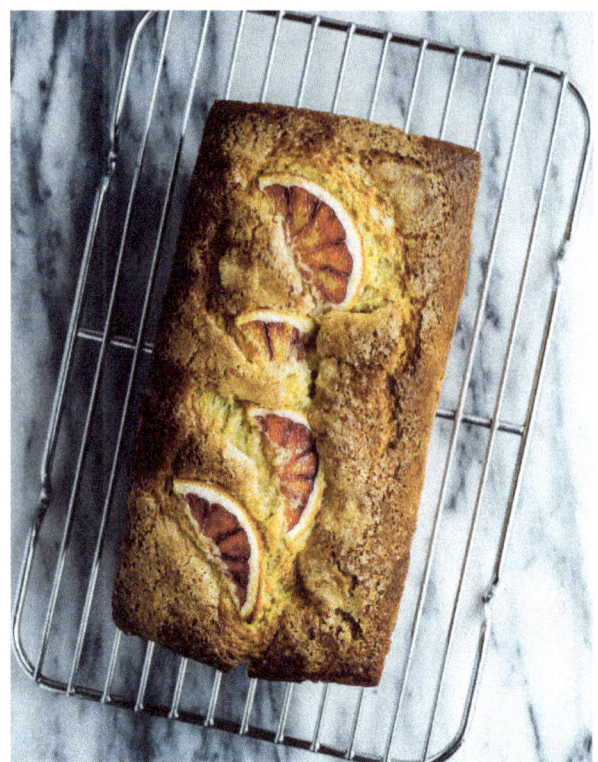

INGREDIENTS

- Cooking splash or extra-virgin olive oil
- 1 medium blood orange
- 1/4 cups generally useful flour
- 1/2 cup medium-crush cornmeal
- 2 teaspoons preparing powder
- 1/4 teaspoon preparing pop
- 1/4 teaspoon fine salt
- 2/3 cup in addition to 2 tablespoons granulated sugar, separated
- 1/2 cup entire milk plain yogurt
- 3 huge eggs
- 1/2 cup extra-virgin olive oil

- 4 paper-slim half-moon-formed blood orange cuts (discretionary)

Process:

Orchestrate a rack in the broiler and warmth to 350°F. Oil a 9-by 5-inch portion skillet with cooking splash or oil; put in a safe spot. Utilizing a vegetable peeler, eliminate the zing from the orange. Cut the zing into slender strips and put in a safe spot. Juice the orange and put aside 1/4 cup (save the leftover juice for utilization). Whisk the flour, cornmeal, heating powder, preparing pop, and salt together in a medium bowl; put in a safe spot. Whisk 2/3 cup of the sugar and the 1/4 cup blood orange squeeze together in enormous bowl. Each in turn, speeds in the yogurt, eggs, and olive oil. Whisk the flour combination into the wet ingredients, giving the blend 20 great turns with the speed until just joined. Overlap in the zing strips. Move the hitter into the readied skillet. Top with the blood orange cuts and staying 2 tablespoons sugar. Heat until the top is springy and brilliant earthy colored, and a wooden stick embedded in the middle comes out with only a couple morsels joined, 50 to an hour. Allow the cake to cool in the dish on a wire rack for 20 minutes. Cautiously unmold the cake, flip it back to be straight up, and get back to the rack to cool totally.

69. Honeyed Phyllo Stacks with Pistachios, Spiced Fruit & Yogurt

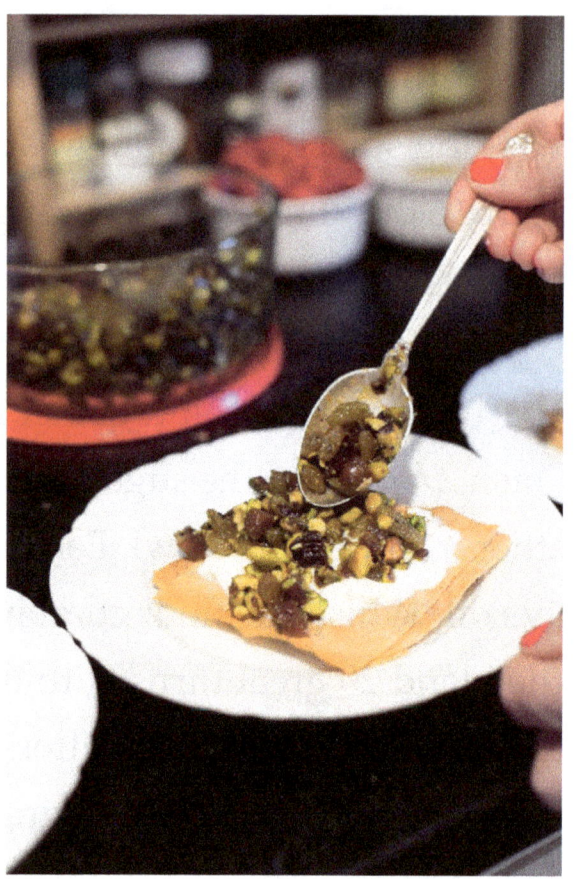

INGREDIENTS

- For the phyllo mixture:
- 6 sheets phyllo mixture, defrosted
- 1/4 cup sugar
- 1/4 teaspoon ground cinnamon
- 1/4 cup extra-virgin olive oil
- For the pistachio and organic product blend:
- Zing and juice of 1 orange (around 1/4 cup juice)
- 2 tablespoons sugar
- 2 tablespoons nectar

- 1/2 cup dried brilliant raisins, generally cleaved
- 1 cup cooked unsalted pistachio nuts, generally cleaved
- 1/2 cup pitted dates, generally cleaved
- 1/2 teaspoon ground cardamom

For yogurt:
- 1 cup entire milk Greek yogurt
- 1 tablespoon confectioners' sugar
- Zing of 1 lemon

For serving:
- 1/2 cup pomegranate arils
- 1/4 cup pistachios, cleaved
- Nectar, warmed
- Raspberries or strawberries to decorate, discretionary

Process:

To set up the phyllo squares:

Preheat the broiler to 400°F and fix an enormous preparing sheet with material. Stack the phyllo sheets on the ledge and cover freely with a scarcely soggy towel. Join the sugar and cinnamon in a little bowl. Put the oil in another little bowl. Eliminate a sheet of phyllo and spot it on the readied preparing sheet. Utilizing a cake brush, gently cover the phyllo mixture with the olive oil and sprinkle softly with the cinnamon sugar. Top with another sheet of phyllo, oil, and cinnamon sugar. Rehash with the entirety of the sheets, yet when you get to the top layer, brushes it gently with oil. Use kitchen shears to clip the layered mixture into 12 squares or square shapes of equivalent size. Heat the phyllo batter for 7 to 8 minutes or until it is brilliant earthy colored and fresh. Allow it to cool totally. The readied phyllo squares can be put away in a water/air proof holder at room temperature for as long as 3 days.

For pistachio and fruit mix:

In a little pot, heat the orange zing and orange squeeze, sugar, and nectar until the juice boils and the nectar breaks down. Mix in the brilliant raisins and put the dish in a safe spot. Blend the pistachios in with the dates. Mix in the cardamom. Mix the spiced pistachios and dates into the container with the syrup and raisins. Put aside the pistachio and organic product blend to marinate for in any event 30 minutes. This combination can be made as long as 5 days early and put away in the fridge.

For yogurt:

Altogether blend the yogurt in with the confectioners' sugar and lemon zing. The yogurt combination can be refrigerated for as long as 5 days, all around covered.

For dessert:

Smear around 1 tablespoon of yogurt on a phyllo cake square. Spot on an individual dessert plate. Top with a liberal spoonful of the organic product combination, at that point another phyllo square. Rehash, and top with a last cake square and a little dab of yogurt. Sprinkle the stack and the dish around it with pomegranate arils and pistachios; at that point shower delicately with warmed nectar. Rehash, making 4 phyllo square stacks, and serve right away. Enhancement whenever wanted with occasional organic product like raspberries or strawberries.

70. Aztec Chocolate Granola Bark

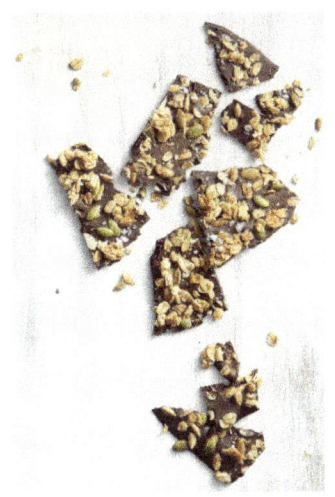

Ingredients:

8 oz. dark chocolate, chopped

1 c. Sweet and Spicy Granola

1/2 tsp. flaky sea salt

Process:

Melt dark chocolate on flame, stirring every 15 seconds until completely melted and smooth. Spread onto parchment in 9- by 14-inch rectangle. Scatter Sweet and Spicy Granola over chocolate and sprinkle with flaky sea salt. Refrigerate until set, about 20 minutes. Break into pieces to serve. Can be refrigerated up to 1 week.

The 15-Day Women's Health Book of 15-Minute Workouts

The Time-Saving Program to Raise a Leaner, Stronger, More Muscular You

Anphora Cooper

Table of Contents

Introduction	**158**
Chapter 1: What is the 15-Minute workouts?	**160**
WORK SMARTER, NOT HARDER	160
A HEALTHIER LIFESTYLE	161
ALL YOU NEED IS YOU	162
Chapter 2: The Science of Leanness	**164**
LEANNESS IS NOT A FOUR-LETTER WORD	165
DIET	166
DIETING TIPS	167
Chapter 3: How to Maximize Post-Workout Recovery so You Can Train Harder and Recover Faster.	**171**
MAXIMIZING POST-WORKOUT RECOVERY	174
Chapter 4: The Science of Muscular Strength	**176**
MUSCULAR STRENGTH AND DEVELOPMENT FACTS	176
HOW THE BODY CREATES MUSCLE	178
Chapter 5: How to Build Lean Muscle (and Raise Your Metabolism)	**180**
SAMPLE WORKOUT SCHEDULE	183
DAY 1: CHEST/TRICEPS (REST DAY)	184
DAY 2: BACK/BICEPS (REST DAY)	185
DAY 3: LEGS/CORE(REST DAY)	186
DAY 4: CHEST/TRICEPS (REST DAY)	187
DAY 5: BACK/BICEPS (REST DAY)	188
Chapter 6: Resize Your Thighs	**191**

LEG AND THIGH WORKOUT 1 — 191
  PART A — 191
  PART B — 193
LEG AND THIGH WORKOUT 2 — 195
LOWER BODY WORKOUT 3 — 197
LEG AND THIGH WORKOUT 4 — 198
  PART A — 198
  PART B — 198
LEG AND THIGH WORKOUT 5 — 199

Chapter 7: The Lean 15-Minute Workouts for Building Muscle and Losing Fat — 200

Chapter 8: The 15-Day Body of Your Dreams in Just 15 Minutes a Day (or Less) — 206

PART I. INTRODUCTION TO THE 15 DAY LEAN BODY PROGRAM — 206
PART II. THE FAST TRACK TO THE CORE PROGRAM — 209
PART III. THE FAST TRACK TO THE FAT BURN PROGRAM — 211
PART IV. WRAPPING UP WITH FAT-BURNING TIPS FROM OUR ALL-STAR TEAM — 213

Chapter 9: Benefits Of 15 Minutes Workout — 216

THERE ARE VARIOUS TIPS WHICH NEEDS TO BE FOLLOWED BEFORE EXERCISING — 216

Conclusion — 222

Introduction

The 15-Day Fast Track to the Core Program is exactly that...a program that walks you step by step through a 15-minute workout template designed to take your body from a fat-storing machine into a lean, mean, calorie burning machine. OK, so you don't burn calories while sleeping or when you're sitting at your desk, but when you are exercising vigorously like in the 15-Minute Workout, you torch calories and fat at an accelerated rate. The program is designed to get the most out of each workout session by working every muscle group with tri-sets and supersets. The tri-sets and supersets are done so that you are constantly changing the angle of your muscles and joints. This keeps the workout from getting tedious and monotonous. It also increases your metabolism, thus preventing you from getting bored with the workouts.

This program is also designed to be as easy as possible in regard to equipment. I have tried my best to build a program that requires no equipment at all, or if you do have equipment, it should be simple and easy to get your hands on if you don't already own it. The only equipment you need is a set of dumbbells, though I do highly suggest you use a core stabilization ball and a resistance band. You can go to any department store and pick up these items, or if you are like me, your local grocery store has these readily available. The way I look at it is that if they sell it in the grocery store, then it must be pretty good for me! Now before we get into the program itself, I want to give you some tips on what to do with your day between workout sessions. We're not going to make our workouts longer but we will make them more productive by adding just two minutes of cardio work between the warm-up and cool-down period. This will help you burn more fat and calories throughout the day in between your workout sessions. How do I know what to do? Well, a lot of the things I have learned about working out is by studying bodybuilders. Bodybuilders aren't just people who want to be big and bulky...they also must have an incredible degree of muscular definition. The reason for this is that they are judged by how ripped their muscles are as well as how big they are when it comes to competitions such as the Mr. and Miss shows or Mr. Olympia! Bodybuilders know that if you wanted to win, you needed every muscle fibre in your body working together and functioning at its maximum capacity all the time. The only way you can do this is by having some sort of cardiovascular training done daily.

Chapter 1: What is the 15-Minute workouts?

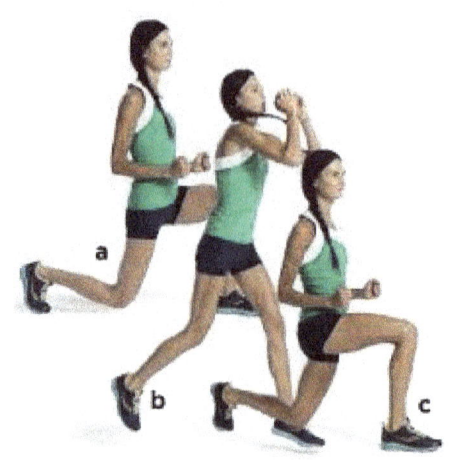

Work Smarter, Not Harder

Every second counts during your busy day—which is why you need a workout program that doesn't take up any of your precious minutes. So we asked our Men's Health Personal Trainer of the Year, Rachel Cosgrove, co-owner of Results Fitness in California and one of the country's top trainers, to create a fast workout routine for women. This 15-day plan will get you looking and feeling better fast.

Each day's workout targets a specific body part and burns about 400 calories. That's an extra 400 calories burned each day, just like that. And, since you're only doing 15 minutes at a time, you can squeeze in these workouts anytime—no excuses! This plan is designed to be easy to follow at home or at the gym. You'll do seven supersets—a superset is when you alternate one set of an exercise with one set of another, back and forth without resting in between. The only rest you get is when it says REST (about a minute). Cosgrove will show you how it works in the video above.

Targeted Training for Busy Women

Each day's workout targets a specific body part with the goal of burning 400 calories. Example: If you do the plan on Monday and Wednesday, your week will be broken down as such: Monday—legs day and upper back day; Wednesday—arms and abs. This allows you to target your hard-to-tone trouble spots in just 15 minutes a day! The workouts are designed to be performed at home or at the gym. You'll do seven supersets—a superset is when you alternate one set of an exercise with one set of another, back and forth without resting in between.

A Healthier Lifestyle

Adding more exercise to your life can only benefit you, provided you exercise safely as discussed in more detail in the next chapter. However, if you are working out to lose weight in addition to becoming more physically fit, you will need to make changes to your diet as well.

The 15-Minute Body Fix will work best when accompanied by these changes. Observing portion sizes, choosing foods that are more nutritious, and limiting sugar, starch and alcohol will improve your health and the effectiveness of your workout.

Be aware, it's not necessary to change radically all aspects of your life at once. In fact, this can sabotage your plans before you really get started by overwhelming your system. Add elements of the 15-Minute Body Fix gradually to your life, and continue adding consistently until you are meeting your final goal.

All You Need Is You

A common complaint about beginning a fitness routine is expense: extensive equipment and videos to buy, or a pricey gym membership. All the workouts in the 15-Minute Body Fix are specifically chose to require little more equipment than your body weight.

Body weight workouts are designed to use your own weight instead of a dumbbell. These kinds of exercises place your body in what is called a disadvantaged position, requiring more strength to make the move. Pushups are the most famous of these exercises, but there are many more. These workouts also usually require the use of several muscle groups, so even if they are zone targeted, you will still continue to strengthen your other parts.

If any other equipment is involved, it will be a common household item, like a towel or a chair. You may also need to use a wall stabilize yourself. You will need a timer. However, a common kitchen timer will do, as will the stopwatch function on most cell phones. No fancy fitness equipment is needed for the 15-Minute Body Fix.

Chapter 2: The Science of Leanness

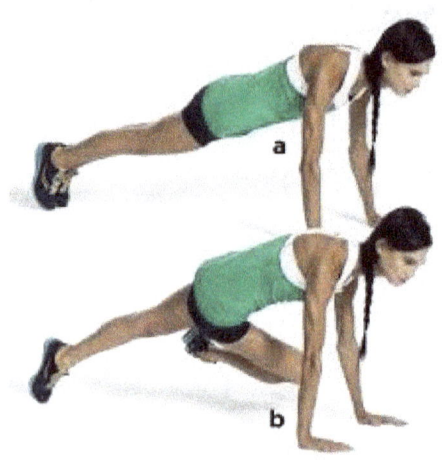

This is the most important chapter in the book. This chapter will teach you everything you need to know about how the human body burns fat and how you can rev up your metabolism so it's operating at its maximum efficiency even if you're not working out. I will also be covering a condition called insulin resistance which is a condition that slows down your metabolism and makes it harder for your body to burn fat. The good news is that insulin resistance is preventable by making small changes in everyday life. It's not something you just have to live with. You will find that in this program, the majority of your workouts focus around the muscles in the core area. The reason for this is because the core is considered to be one of the most important areas for increasing calorie burning. I will also be teaching you how to rev up your metabolism with some simple but very effective exercises. To top it off, I'm also going to teach you about what and when to eat so that you can get all of the fat-burning benefits possible out of your diet plan!

Leanness Is NOT a Four-Letter Word

We have to change the way we look at fat and leanness in the modern day. The fitness world has made us think that being "fat" is something to be ashamed of and that putting on lean muscle is something that you have to work forever for. I'm here to tell you that this is simply not true! It's not true because all of us have fat on our bodies. We need fat to survive! It is true that our bodies can become much healthier if we have more lean muscle on our bodies and less fat but that's not the key. The key is getting leaner while preserving as much muscle tissue as possible. There are some people out there who believe that it's easier to lose weight by burning off as much of the muscle tissue as possible while you're going on a diet. The reason some people think this way is because they are always hungry and they feel lethargic. This is a complete lie! The easiest way to lose weight and keep your muscles intact is to consume just enough nutrients so you don't lose any muscle mass while losing body fat. If you consume an extreme amount of lean protein and just the right amount of carbohydrates, your body will enter a state called ketosis which is a state in which your body burns fat for energy instead of carbohydrates. The only time that carbs are burned is during intense exercise like sprinting. This mean that if you're at a standstill, your body is going to burn fat for energy instead of carbs. Keep in mind that this approach to getting leaner has to be done with long-term consistency. You cannot do this program once every two months and expect to see good results. You can only get the good results by making small changes to your daily life and doing it consistently over time. The worst thing that you can do is to try this program for 3 days and then quit. If you do that, all the time and money that you spent on your supplements will have been a waste. Over the next few sections, I'm going to teach you everything that I have learned over the past 12 years about losing fat while keeping muscle.

Diet

I would like to say it straight out the gate…"There is no quick fix diet!" There are some people who may lose fat quickly but those people are not eating healthy either. Just because you aren't hungry doesn't mean it isn't hurting your body. You will not get the best results with those crazy 3 day diets that you see on TV. Also, if there was a quick fix to losing fat, I could be gone by now. I would have already made my millions and wouldn't be writing these messages to you. There is no magic diet pill or potion that will make it easy for you to lose fat. The old adage "you can't out train a bad diet" cannot be put any more accurately than it is in this sentence. A good diet plays a significant role in getting leaner or building muscle because it is used as the source for your energy (calories) for your body to burn off of. If you don't have the proper nutrients coming in from your diet, your body is going to be forced to tap into muscles and fat tissue for energy. So having a good diet is a must for everyone, no matter what his or her goals may be.

Dieting Tips

1) Cut your portions- The easiest way to start decreasing the amount of calories that you are taking in is to simply cut your portion sizes down. Most people tend to eat overly large portions that main reason being that people cannot deal with having food go away on their plates. If you take in a large portion and finish it all, you feel accomplished. If the food that you ate was low calorie, then there shouldn't be anything to feel accomplished about. So I suggest taking your regular plate of food and half the size so that you're consuming less calories at each sitting. After the first week or two, get another plate of half the size and half with your original sized plate which will now be your medium sized plate. This will help

you get into a routine of eating smaller portions by simply changing out your plates.

2) Eat more often- With the first tip, we want to start becoming in tune with our body's natural hunger signals. We can do this by simply eating more often. I suggest eating 4 meals a day, and 2 snacks. How you eat is not important as long as you are eating smaller portions and getting enough nutrients each day. As I will discuss in my nutrition plan, your meals should consist of a lean protein, fibre filled carbohydrate and a low glycemic index (low sugar) carbohydrate. This is just the basic outline for eating. As we get into the plan in the next few sections, I am going to tell you exactly what to eat for each meal.

3) Avoid sweeteners- Many people turn to sweeteners in order to cut calories from their diet and still have dessert. These sweeteners are usually found in desserts and beverages like soda or juice with little or no real nutritional value. These types of foods will sabotage your efforts because you will simply fill up on them while not getting enough nutrients in your body. The best thing to do is avoid these types of foods all together. This may sound like it's impossible but if you just put in a little extra effort into planning your meals ahead of time, you will find that it's really not that hard and you will actually be able to enjoy more variety in your diet. I'm not

suggesting that you have to cut out desserts for the rest of your life but what I am saying is that if you are trying to get leaner, then it doesn't make any sense at all to eat something that is going to sabotage your efforts.

4) Avoid Sodium- You may have heard this before...but sodium makes us retain water. If you are retaining water, it makes it look like you're not losing fat because your muscles are not as defined as they could be. So this is another area where you need to cut corners. Salt your food sparingly and find a low sodium sports drink or water if you are out and about. If you don't have time to prepare your own meals, try finding restaurants that serve mainly seafood or eat at home. It's much easier for them to control their sodium levels than other types of restaurants.

5) Take your vitamins- Many times, when people go on a diet, they tend to forget about their vitamins and multivitamins. You should always take them even if you are eating a healthy diet. Vitamins and minerals are what make up muscles so without them, you will be losing weight from your muscles instead of fat. A fat loss and muscle building supplement is also a good option for you to use if you just aren't getting enough nutrients in your body each day (I will discuss this in my nutrition plan).

6) Keep Hydrated- I'm sure you've heard this many times but it's important so I'll say it again...Keep Hydrated! You should shoot for at least 8 glasses of water a day. Most people get all of their water from drinks like soda or juice which are just sugar water with no nutritional value what so ever.

7) Get Enough Sleep- I have already discussed how important sleep is in making muscle gains but another big reason why it's important is because your metabolism is highest when you're sleeping. This means that you should be getting enough sleep each night. If you're only sleeping 5 hours per night, then try to get more by either going to bed earlier or waking up later in the morning.

Chapter 3: How to Maximize Post-Workout Recovery so You Can Train Harder and Recover Faster.

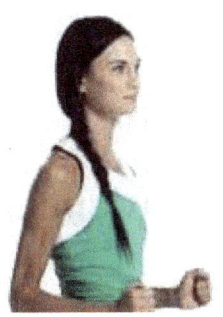

If you want to build a lean and muscular body, you have to train hard and often. Training hard is one thing if you can recover quickly, but if your muscles have a difficult time recovering after a heavy weight training session then all your hard work will be for nothing.

The goal of this chapter is to show you exactly what foods and supplements you can use to help your body recover fast from exercise.

1) Eat smart before going to bed- Try eating more the night before so that you wake up with an empty stomach (don't eat within 3 hours of going to sleep). Make sure your last meal before bed consists of mostly protein. This will help your body repair and recover from weight training while you sleep.

2) Sleep long enough- Not getting enough sleep is the main reason why people can't recover from exercise, because you body needs

rest and recuperation. The average person should get between 7-9 hours of sleep per night.

3) Eat protein every 3-4 hours while awake- If you wake up at 6am, try eating a snack that consists of protein like a piece or two of chicken or drink whey protein (depending on your schedule). Then, eat a main meal that consists of a protein source like steak or chicken with a carbohydrate source. Then, have another snack that consists of protein like whey protein or a piece of deli turkey an hour or so after you eat your meal. Then, have another meal an hour after you have your snack and then eat dinner quite late at night (this way you will wake up with an empty stomach). Also, make sure to drink plenty of water to stay hydrated. If you are unable to eat every 3-4 hours while awake then take some type of protein supplement that uses slow-digesting proteins for long lasting amino acid delivery (whey is fast-digesting, casein is slow-digesting).

4) Take supplements- I would recommend taking some type of protein supplement before, during, and after exercise. You can use whey protein, casein protein, milk proteins (such as Optimum Nutrition 100% Whey Gold Standard), etc. I would also recommend using a multivitamin every day as well as 6-8 grams of BCAA's before and after exercise (I take Optimum Nutrition Amino Energy

due to the fact that it contains creatine monohydrate). I recommend using creatine monohydrate because it has been proven to increase strength and lean muscle tissue over a period of time when taken consistently.

5) Eat regularly- Eating many small meals throughout the day is better for recovery than eating a few big meals.

6) Eat more fruits and vegetables- Fruits and vegetables contain important micronutrients that are important for recovery. Also, fruits and vegetables contain carbohydrates which you can absorb quickly to replenish muscle glycogen stores.

7) Eat healthy fats- Healthy fats such as olive oil, coconut oil, flaxseed oil, avocados, nuts, etc. help your body absorb the fat soluble vitamins A,D, E and K from the foods you eat.

8) Drink milk- Milk contains both slow-digesting proteins (casein) and fast-digesting proteins (whey). This makes milk a great post workout supplement.

9) Drink alcohol moderately- Drinking a glass of red wine daily has been shown to improve recovery from exercise.

10) Drink coffee- Research has shown that the amino acid L-Carnitine is found in higher levels in people who drink coffee compared to people who don't drink it. This is important because L-

Carnitine helps transport fatty acids into the mitochondria of muscle cells so that they can be used as fuel for energy. The more fatty acids you can get into your mitochondria, the more fat you will burn throughout the day. Also, caffeine in coffee stimulates your central nervous system to make it easy for you to wake up and become highly alert.

Maximizing Post-Workout Recovery

Here is the list of foods and supplements that will help maximize post workout recovery:

1. Lean meats like chicken, turkey, and beef as well as fish

2. Eggs

3. Plant based protein powders

4. Whole milk

5. Whey protein powders (fast absorbing)

6. Casein protein powders (slow absorbing)

7. Multivitamins- Look for ones that contain calcium, magnesium, zinc, B vitamins, vitamin D3 (cholecalciferol), etc...

8. BCAA supplements- Drink these before and after training.

9. Creatine monohydrate

10. Caffeine from coffee or green tea

11. Fruits and vegetables

12. Healthy fats like olive oil, avocados, nuts, fatty fish (e.g., salmon), etc...

13. Milk- Consume this right after you train because it has both fast-digesting whey protein as well as slow-digesting casein protein in it (whey is fast digesting; casein is slow digesting).

14. Alcohol in moderation (e.g., 1 glass of red wine a day) has been shown to improve recovery from exercise .

Chapter 4: The Science of Muscular Strength

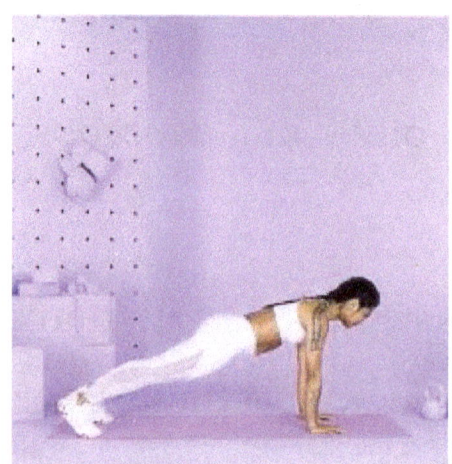

This chapter will teach you everything you need to know about building muscle. I'm not going to be teaching you how to do hundreds of different exercises. Instead, I'm going to be teaching you the most effective compound exercises (multi-joint) for each body part in terms of developing overall strength and increasing lean muscle mass. You will notice that there is a lot of attention paid towards your core muscles. Your core muscles are considered to be the most important muscle group in your body because they play a significant role in stabilizing your spine and increasing calorie burning. I will also be teaching you the different types of muscle fibres and how they help your body in everyday activities. Understanding how muscles work will help you to know what you need to do in order to build strength and muscle.

Muscular Strength and Development Facts

1) There are 2 types of muscle fibres found in our bodies. These are known as Type 1 and Type 2 muscle fibres. There is a simple way to remember them...Type 1 is called Slow twitch and Type 2 is called Fast Twitch. Slow twitch or Type 1 is designed for endurance, whereas fast Twitch or Type 2's main function is power. Slow twitch fibres burn more calories than fast twitch fibres which make them the best choice for your body when it comes to losing fat while preserving as much muscle as possible.

2) In order to build strength and aesthetics, you need to focus on compound exercises that work the major muscle groups of your body. Compound exercises are multijoint exercises (exercises that involve more than one major body part) that use large, powerful movements in order to help your body develop overall strength. These are going to be the exercises that I will be focusing on for you over the next few chapters.

3) Whenever you feel fatigued during an exercise, it is usually a sign that you should stop the exercise and not push through with prolonged muscle failure. Prolonged muscle failure can cause your muscles to have delayed onset muscle soreness (DOMS) as well as take longer for your muscles to repair and rebuild themselves.

4) In order to build strength and muscle, you must eat enough calories and protein. Calories are the basic building blocks of energy needed for your muscles to repair themselves after an intense workout. Protein not only builds your muscles but it also helps them retain water which gives you a pumped look. I will discuss all of these nutrients as we get into my nutrition plan later on in this book.

5) Although I said that slow twitch fibres are more efficient for burning calories, they do not have the ability to explode or generate as much power as fast twitch fibres can. This is why you need to use both types of exercises in order to develop strength and aesthetics (looks).

How The Body Creates Muscle

The task of strength and muscle development can be very complicated. I'm not going to get into the details of it, but I will give you a brief overview of what is happening during a typical muscle building process.

As we begin to lift heavy weights, two important reactions take place in the body. The first is that the brain releases a chemical known as adrenaline (epinephrine). Adrenaline speeds up the heart rate and makes more blood available for muscular contraction. This reaction increases muscular strength which is needed as your body begins to lift heavier weights. This reaction occurs for only a short period of time in order to maximize your ability to lift while not overworking your body.

The second reaction, which can last up to 48 hours after a rigorous workout session, is when your body releases growth hormone (GH). During this time, GH stimulates the muscles to repair themselves as quickly as possible. This allows your body to build more muscle for future workouts. GH is also responsible for the burning sensation you feel 24-48 hours later.

In order to develop strength and increase lean muscle mass, you need to keep challenging your body by upping the intensity of your workouts. Your body will adapt within 3-4 weeks if you are training properly and doing more than just lifting light weights with poor form. You must keep your brain thinking that you're not capable of handling the amount of weight you are lifting if you want to continue to make progress.

Chapter 5: How to Build Lean Muscle (and Raise Your Metabolism)

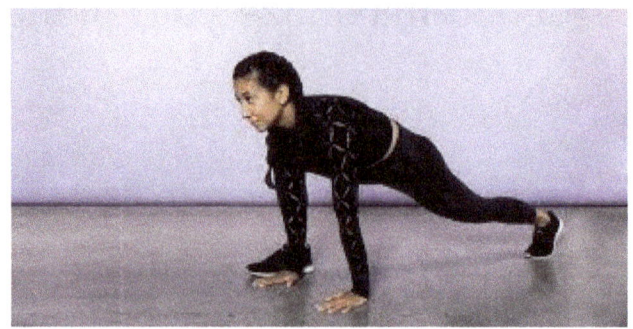

This chapter will be all about developing lean muscle mass. I will be discussing the six steps to building muscle and the type of equipment you should be using for each step. I will also give you a sample workout schedule to follow at the end. The first step to building muscle is stretching which I will discuss in this chapter as well.

I'm going to start by talking about how important it is for your muscles to stretch before and after every workout you do (this includes stretching your core). The main reason why it's important is because if you stretch the muscles, tendons and ligaments before a workout, then they are much more apt to being stretched during the workout as well. If you stretch before a workout, then your body will be much more flexible and better capable of handling the stress of your weight training. Lifting weights puts a lot of pressure on the muscles that you are exercising. If you don't stretch before your workout, then the pressure on those muscles can cause them to tighten up and become very stiff which can result in muscle strains. I'm sure you know what this feels like from either experience or just seeing someone else with a muscle pull while working out. This is also known as delayed onset muscle soreness (DOMS) which I will discuss later on.

Understand that all of your workouts should be done in a progressive manner which means that each workout gets more intense than the last and that the weight you are using increases every week. There are six steps to developing lean muscle mass. These steps include: stretching, dynamic flexibility, active flexibility, traditional strength training, pre-exhaustion and super sets. Here they are in more detail:

1) Stretching- Before doing any kind of weight training or flexibility exercises, you need to stretch for at least 10 minutes or until you feel completely stretched out. When doing this stretch routine, make sure to hold each stretch for 15 seconds before moving on to the next one (I'll discuss how to do each stretch later).

Stretching will do two things for you. First of all, it will improve your flexibility which is needed in order to perform some of the exercises I'll be teaching you. Secondly, it will help to keep your muscles from becoming tight which can result from being under too much stress while weight training (I explained how this works in the "Building Lean Mass" chapter).

2) Dynamic Flexibility- Dynamic flexibility is very similar to static stretching except that dynamic flexibility incorporates movement into the stretch so that you are actually moving through your range of motion. This type of stretching should also be done before your weight training workouts as well. The best way to do this is to start by loosening up your muscles and then move through your range of motion as you would when doing the actual exercise. I'll demonstrate this in more detail later on.

3) Active Flexibility- Active flexibility is basically doing the opposite of static stretching. Instead of holding a stretch for 15 seconds, you're going to hold it for 15 seconds or however long you can before your muscles begin to tighten back up and then contract yourself for 15 seconds (this applies when doing crunches or sit ups). This type of stretching should also be done before each workout session, especially lower body days.

4) Traditional Strength Training- This is what most people think of when they hear the words "weight training". This is where you use heavy weights and perform an exercise in a controlled manner in

order to develop the strength of that particular muscle. You should use between 3-5 sets per exercise and do 4-6 repetitions for each set. When you are doing these exercises, don't just lift the weight up and down without any control. You should be using your muscles to move the weight up and down. If you are just moving sluggishly through your range of motion then it means that you aren't getting a good workout.

5) Pre-Exhaust Training- Here you will be doing a set of an exercise for one particular muscle group and then immediately (with no rest in between) doing a set of an exercise that works the same muscle group but with a different range of motion. This is considered to be one superset. This is another way to challenge your body so that it continually adapts to the stress you are putting on it.

6) Super Sets- Here you will be doing two exercises for the same muscle group without any rest in between them. You should do each super set for 3 sets per exercise and 6 repetitions per set (I'll explain how to choose the right amount weight later).

Sample Workout Schedule

I am going to give you a sample workout schedule that you can try. This is a six day per week split routine and will involve several strength training exercises as well as active flexibility, dynamic flexibility and stretching for each muscle group. The first four days will be for training your upper body and the last two days will be for your lower body. It's important that you change up the order of these workouts every other week at least so that your body doesn't adapt to the workout routine repetition. Before each workout, warm up for 10-15 minutes by either doing some cardio or jogging in place (I will discuss warming up in more detail later on).

This schedule should be used as an example for you to follow and not as a "set in stone" plan. You need to change it up each time to make sure your body doesn't adapt to the same workout routine.

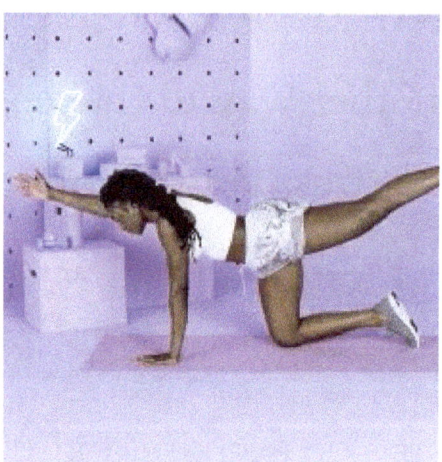

Day 1: Chest/Triceps (Rest Day)

A. Barbell Bench Press 3 x 8-12 reps

B. Cable Crossover 2 x 15-20 reps

C. Chest Stretch 5-10 reps (hold for 15 seconds)

D. Triceps Stretch (active flexibility) 5-10 reps (hold for 15 seconds)

E. Triceps Stretch (static flexibility) 10-15 reps

F. Clasping Triceps Stretch 10-15 reps

G. Clasping Rear Delt Stretch 10-15 reps

H. Chest Stretch 5-10 reps (hold for 15 seconds)

I. Triceps Stretch (active flexibility) 5-10 reps (hold for 15 seconds)

J. Triceps Stretch (static flexibility) 10-15 reps

K. Clasping Triceps Stretch 10-15 reps

L. Clasping Rear Delt Stretch 5-10 reps

M. Active Back Flexibility Workout (details later)

Day 2: Back/Biceps (Rest Day)

A. Barbell Deadlift 3 x 8-12 reps

B. Seated Row 3 x 8-12 reps

C. Lat Stretch 5-10 reps (hold for 15 seconds)

D. Bicep Stretch (active flexibility) 5-10 reps (hold for 15 seconds)

E. Bicep Stretch (static flexibility) 10-15 reps

F. Kneeling Overhead Triceps Stretch 10-15 reps

G. Head to Toe Bicep Stretch 10-15 reps

H. Lat Stretch 5-10 reps (hold for 15 seconds)

I. Bicep Stretch (active flexibility) 5-10 reps (hold for 15 seconds)

J. Bicep Stretch (static flexibility) 10-15 reps

K. Kneeling Overhead Triceps Stretch 10-15 reps

L. Head to Toe Bicep Stretch 10-15 reps

M. Lat Stretch 5-10 reps (hold for 15 seconds)

N. Bicep Stretch (active flexibility) 5-10 reps (hold for 15 seconds)

O. Bicep Stretch (static flexibility) 10-15 reps

P. Kneeling Overhead Triceps Stretch 10-15 reps

Q. Head to Toe Bicep Stretch 10-15 reps

Day 3: Legs/Core(Rest Day)

A. Barbell Deadlift 3 x 8-12 reps

B. Leg Press 3 x 8-12 reps

C. Cable Woodchop 2 x 15-20 reps

D. Hip Flexor Stretch 5-10 reps (hold for 15 seconds; each leg)

E. Hamstring Stretch (active flexibility) 5-10 reps (hold for 15 seconds; each leg)

F. Hamstring Stretch (static flexibility) 10-15 reps

G. Quad Stretch 5-10 reps (hold for 15 seconds; each leg)

H. Lat Stretch 5-10 reps (hold for 15 seconds; each leg)

I. Bicep Stretch (active flexibility) 5-10 reps (hold for 15 seconds; each arm)

J. Bicep Stretch (static flexibility) 10-15 reps

K. Kneeling Overhead Triceps Stretch 10-15 reps

L. Clasping Triceps Stretch 10-15 reps

M. Clasping Rear Delt Stretch 5-10 reps

N. Core Flexibility Workout (details later)

Day 4: Chest/Triceps (Rest Day)

A. Flat Barbell Bench Press 3 x 8-12 reps

B. Decline Push Up 2 x 15-20 reps

C. Chest Stretch 5-10 reps (hold for 15 seconds)

D. Tricep Stretch (active flexibility) 5-10 reps (hold for 15 seconds)

E. Tricep Stretch (static flexibility) 10-15 reps

F. Clasping Tricep Stretch 10-15 reps

G. Clasping Rear Delt Stretch 10-15 reps

H. Chest Stretch 5-10 reps (hold for 15 seconds)

I. Tricep Stretch (active flexibility) 5-10 reps (hold for 15 seconds)

J. Tricep Stretch (static flexibility) 10-15 reps

K. Clasping Tricep Stretch 10-15 reps

L. Clasping Rear Delt Stretch 5-10 reps

M. Active Back Flexibility Workout (details later)

Day 5: Back/Biceps (Rest Day)

A. Good Morning 3 x 8-12 reps

B. Deadlift 3 x 8-12 reps

C. Lat Stretch 5-10 reps (hold for 15 seconds; each arm)

D. Bicep Stretch (active flexibility) 5-10 reps (hold for 15 seconds; each arm)

E. Bicep Stretch (static flexibility) 10-15 reps

F. Kneeling Overhead Tricep Stretch 10-15 reps

G. Clasping Front Delt Stretch 10-15 reps

H. Lat Stretch 5-10 reps (hold for 15 seconds; each arm)

I. Bicep Stretch (active flexibility) 5-10 reps (hold for 15 seconds; each arm)

J. Bicep Stretch (static flexibility) 10-15 reps

K. Kneeling Overhead Tricep Stretch 10-15 reps

L. Clasping Front Delt Stretch 5-10 reps

M. Lat Stretch 5-10 reps (hold for 15 seconds; each arm)

N. Bicep Stretch (active flexibility) 5-10 reps (hold for 15 seconds; each arm)

O. Bicep Stretch (static flexibility) 10-15 reps

P. Kneeling Overhead Tricep Stretch 10-15 reps

Q. Clasping Front Delt Stretch 5-10 reps

R. Lat Stretch 5-10 reps (hold for 15 seconds; each arm)

S. Bicep Stretch (active flexibility) 5-10 reps (hold for 15 seconds; each arm)

T. Bicep Stretch (static flexibility) 10-15 reps

U. Kneeling Overhead Tricep Stretch 10-15 reps

V. Clasping Front Delt Stretch 5-10 reps

W. Lat Stretch 5-10 reps (hold for 15 seconds; each arm)

X. Bicep Stretch (active flexibility) 5-10 reps (hold for 15 seconds; each arm)

Y. Bicep Stretch (static flexibility) 10-15 reps

Z. Kneeling Overhead Tricep Stretch 10-15 reps

AA. Clasping Front Delt Stretch 5-10 reps

BB. Lat Stretch 5-10 reps (hold for 15 seconds; each arm)

CC. Bicep Stretch (active flexibility) 5-10 reps (hold for 15 seconds; each arm)

DD. Bicep Stretch (static flexibility) 10-15 reps

EE. Kneeling Overhead Tricep Stretch 10-15 reps

FF. Clasping Front Delt Stretch 5-10 reps

GG. Lat Stretch 5-10 reps (hold for 15 seconds; each arm)

HH. Bicep Stretch (active flexibility) 5-10 reps (hold for 15 seconds; each arm)

II. Bicep Stretch (static flexibility) 10-15 reps

JJ. Kneeling Overhead Tricep Stretch 10-15 reps

KK. Clasping Front Delt Stretch 5-10 reps

LL. Lat Stretch 5-10 reps (hold for 15 seconds; each arm)

MM. Bicep Stretch (active flexibility) 5-10 reps (hold for 15 seconds; each arm)

Chapter 6: Resize Your Thighs

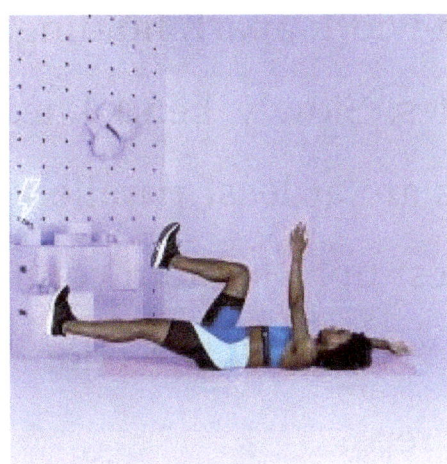

These workouts will focus on your thighs and legs. Although your Full Body Workouts work these muscles, if this is a trouble spot for you in terms of strength, you may want a more targeted routine.

Leg and Thigh Workout 1

This workout is structured as others you have done, organized into Part A and Part B. You will be learning some new exercises, and using some you have already learned.

Part A

Do 10 Squat Jumps are performed safely this way:

Stand with feet together and hands on hips. Keeping your back straight, slowly bend your knees until they are at a 90 degree angle, then thrust upwards, jumping as high as you can. When you land, bring your knees back up to a 90-degree angle. This is one rep.

1. Squats

Stand tall with feet hip-width apart, holding a set of 5- to 15-pound dumbbells at your sides. Slowly bend knees and hips and lower your body until thighs are at least parallel to the floor. Keep head facing forward and chest up. Maintain control of the weights at all times during exercise. Reverse direction to return to starting position and repeat for reps.

2. Lunges

Holding 5- to 15-pound dumbbells in each hand, step forward with left foot and lower body into a lunge until front thigh is parallel to floor; keep back leg straight so that knee does not extend past toe as you go down. Return to start and repeat with right leg. That's 1 rep.

3. Triceps Extensions

Grasp a pair of dumbbells and stand with knees bent and weights hanging at your sides. Straighten arms in front of you until they form a 90-degree angle with your upper arms; keep elbows pointing down toward the floor throughout exercise. Press weights overhead until arms are straight but not locked, then bend elbows to lower them back down. That's 1 rep.

4. Pushups

Start in an elevated pushup position, with hands on the floor directly beneath shoulders, body straight from head to heels, legs extended behind you and toes pointing forward (A). Bend elbows to lower body until chest nearly touches floor (B). Push back up to start and repeat for reps.

5. Squats Alternate with Biceps Curls

Hold a pair of dumbbells in each hand, arms hanging at your sides. Keeping back straight, bend knees and hips as if you were sitting into a chair (A) until thighs are at least parallel to the floor. Now stand and push weights toward ceiling until elbows are fully extended (B). Reverse movement to return to start and repeat for reps.

Do 10 Side Lunges.

Complete Part A 8 times.

Rest 2 minutes.

Part B

Do 10 Jumping Lunges.

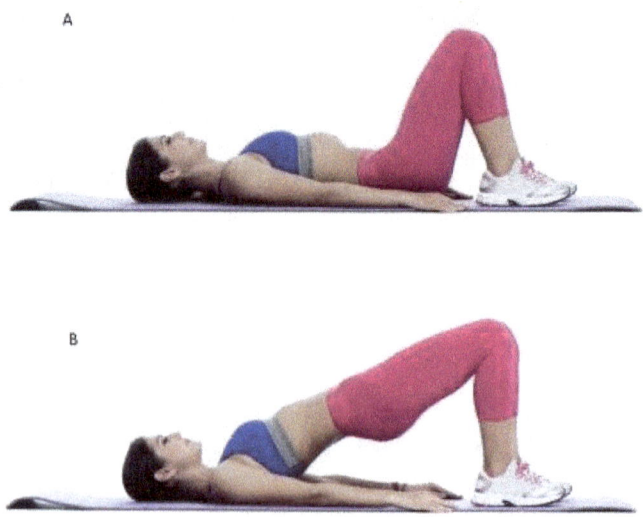

Do 10 Glute Bridges. This is how to do **Glute Bridges:**

1. Lie in neutral position on your back on the floor. A neutral position is not totally flat, nor totally arched. You should be able to slip you hand part way into the curve of your back, but it should not fit all the way.

2. Place your feet, at hip width, evenly on the floor, with your toes pointing forward and your knees bent.

3. Contract your abdominal muscles. Imagine your belly button pulling in toward your spine. Keep your muscles this way throughout the exercise.

4. Push your hips up through your heels. You back should remain in the neutral position. If you back begins to arch or you feel pressure on your neck, you have done too fat.

5. You will keep your abdominals contracted as you lower your hips to the floor.
6. You should not truly rest in between repetitions, only lightly touch the floor.

Complete Part B 8 times.

Rest 2 minutes.

Continue cycling through Parts A and B for 15 minutes.

Leg and Thigh Workout 2

This workout is organized as a circuit. This means that you go from one exercise to another with only a 10 second rest in between. You are measuring by time instead of repetitions, so do each move as quickly and correctly as you can.

Do Squats for 30 seconds

Rest for 10 seconds.

Do Single-Leg Deadlifts for 30 seconds. The **Single-Leg Deadlift** is performed properly this way:

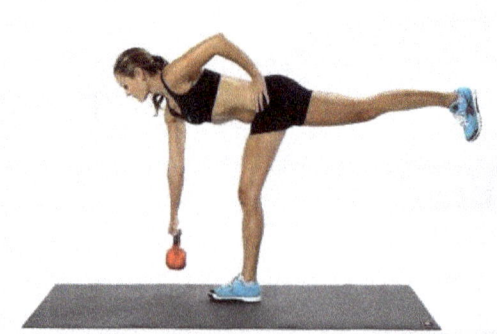

1. Begin in a standing position.
2. Raise one leg straight behind you with your toes pointing downwards.
3. As you raise your leg, bend forward from the hips, keeping your back flat. Keep your neck aligned with your spine, and loose, not tensed.
4. Your hands will be perpendicular to your chest. Do not reach towards the floor, as this may cause you to round your back.
5. Bend only as far as flexibility will allow, while keeping your core tight and your back straight.
6. Continue with your abs tight and your back straight as you lower your leg and return to a standing position.
7. Do not alternate legs until the next circuit. Stick with the single leg.

Rest 10 seconds.

Do Glute Bridges for 30 seconds.

Rest for 1 minute.

Repeat circuit for the entire 15 minutes. If you can only do a few exercises in the 30 seconds, do not get discouraged. You will get faster.

Lower Body Workout 3

This workout follows the pattern, which should now be familiar to you, of 10 repetitions and Jumping Jacks in between.

Begin with 10 Reverse Lunges.

Then do Jumping Jacks until your timer says 1 minute has passed.

At minute 1, do 10 Side Lunges.

Do Jumping Jacks until minute 2.

At minute 2, Do 10 Squats.

Do Jumping Jacks until minute 3.

At minute 3, do 10 Single-Leg Deadlifts.

Do Jumping Jacks until minute 4.

At minute 4, start again.

Do not forget to switch legs on your Single-Leg Deadlifts when you get there.

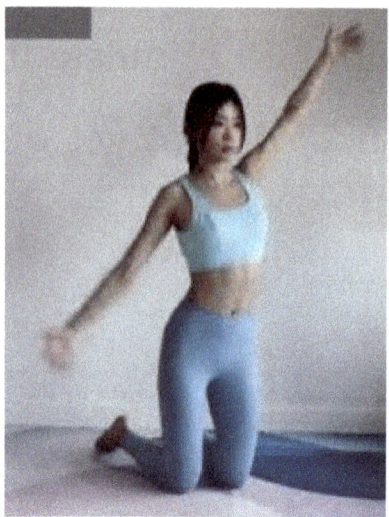

Leg and Thigh Workout 4

This workout will follow the established pattern with Part A and Part B.

Part A

1. Do 10 Jumping Lunges.
2. Rest 10 seconds.
3. Do 10 Single-Leg Deadlifts.
4. Rest 10 seconds.
5. Repeat Part A 8 times.

Part B

1. Do 10 Glute Bridges.
2. Rest 10 seconds.

3. Do 10 Squats.
4. Rest 10 seconds.
5. Repeat Part B 8 times.
6. Cycle between Parts A for the remainder of 15 minutes.

Leg and Thigh Workout 5

This workout is organized as a circuit.

1. Begin with 30 seconds of Jumping Lunges.
2. Rest 10 seconds.
3. Then, do 30 second of Reverse Lunges.
4. Rest 10 seconds.
5. Next, do 30 seconds of Squat Jumps.
6. Rest 1 minute.

Repeat this circuit as many times as you can in 15 minutes.

Chapter 7: The Lean 15-Minute Workouts for Building Muscle and Losing Fat

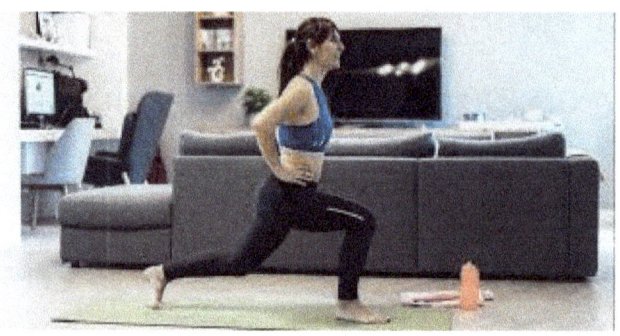

When it comes to building muscle, the biggest obstacle that women face is finding the time to work out. That's why I created The Lean 15 Workouts—the most efficient and effective way for women to burn fat and build lean muscle in only 15 minutes a day. The Lean 15 Workouts take advantage of the body-shaping effects of supersets, which are two exercises performed back-to-back with no rest in between. Supersets force you to work your muscles past their normal failure points, which triggers more growth responses from your body. While you're performing supersets, you'll also be incorporating another muscle-building technique called compound sets, which involve pairing two exercises that work opposing muscle groups. For example, pairing a bench press with a row works your chest and back.

The Lean 15 Workouts employ both of these strategies in dozens of different combinations to help you build and sculpt your entire body. The best part is that each workout keeps your heart rate elevated throughout the entire routine and you only rest when needed—usually between supersets—so you maximize every second of your workout time. The Lean 15 Workouts are divided into two different types of workouts—The Lean 15 Workouts for Beginners and The Lean 15 Workouts for Experienced Exercisers. Below I explain how to use each workout and provide a sample routine that combines exercises from all four phases of the program.

The Lean 15 Workout for Beginners is designed for women who haven't worked out in a while, are new to weight training, or have never lifted weights before. It's also a good option if you've been exercising regularly with moderate intensity but haven't seen any changes in your body or fitness level. The Lean 15 Workout for Beginners will help you build your strength, endurance, and confidence so you can move on to the next phase of the program. The exercises are broken down into four phases—Phase 1: Resistance Training, Phase 2: Strength Training, Phase 3: Advanced Resistance Training and Phase 4: Strength and Power—and each phase works your body in a slightly different way.

In Phase 1: Resistance Training (weeks 1-4), you'll start out with light weights to get used to the exercises and gradually build up your strength. As your muscles get stronger, you'll gradually increase the amount of weight you lift as well as the number of reps you perform. Phase 1: Resistance Training is a great option if you're just starting out with resistance training or you've been working out regularly but haven't seen any changes in your body. Phase 2: Strength Training (weeks 5–8) focuses on increasing the amount of weight you lift for each exercise. To keep your muscles guessing, we incorporate three different supersets—the kickback superset, the press-up superset and the super squat superset—and alternate between them throughout the routine.

The third phase, Phase 3: Advanced Resistance Training (weeks 9–12), builds on the exercises from Phase 2: Strength Training. We also add another superset—this time the single-arm dumbbell row superset—to keep your body working hard. Phase 4: Strength and Power (weeks 13–16) is a repeat of Phase 2: Strength Training. This time, though, you'll be doing many of the exercises for fewer reps and adding more weight to each exercise.

Phases 1: Resistance Training and 2: Strength Training are great options if you've only been exercising for a few weeks or have never lifted weights before. Both phases will help you build strength, endurance and confidence in the gym so you can graduate to the more advanced exercises in Phase 3: Advanced Resistance Training and Phase 4: Strength and Power. The Lean 15 Workout for Experienced Exercisers is designed for women who have been working out regularly with moderate intensity but haven't seen any changes in their body or fitness level. These workouts focus on increasing your weight-training intensity while maintaining the high-energy, fast-paced workouts that I developed for The Lean 15 Workout for Beginners.

For each of the four phases—Phase 1: Resistance Training, Phase 2: Strength Training, Phase 3: Advanced Resistance Training and Phase 4: Strength and Power—you'll perform one set of each exercise in rapid succession with no rest between exercises. Rest only when needed between supersets (usually after you finish a superset). Each phase is slightly different but all four incorporate supersets into the routine. In Phase 1: Resistance Training (weeks 1–4), for example, you'll alternate between two types of supersets—the press-up superset and the kickback superset—and use dumbbells instead of barbells. In Phase 2: Strength Training (weeks 5–8), you'll perform the same exercises as Phase 1: Resistance Training but this time we'll use barbells and alternate between three different supersets —the press-up superset, the single-arm dumbbell row superset and the super squat superset.

In Phase 3: Advanced Resistance Training (weeks 9–12) you'll do the same exercises from Phase 2 but with a third superset—the cable pulldown superset. In Phase 4: Strength and Power (weeks 13–16), we'll take it up a notch by performing many of the exercises for fewer reps and adding more weight to each exercise.

Phase 1: Resistance Training is a great option if you've only been exercising for a few weeks or if you haven't lifted weights before. This phase will help you build confidence and get comfortable with the exercises. Phase 2: Strength Training is a great option if you've been working out regularly but haven't seen any changes in your body or fitness level. Phase 2 not only helps you build strength but also focuses on increasing endurance by alternating between different supersets and adding variety to the exercises.

Phase 3: Advanced Resistance Training focuses on increasing your weight-training intensity while maintaining the high-energy, fast-paced workouts that worked so well in Phases 1 and 2. Phase 4: Strength and Power is for experienced exercisers who have been working out regularly with moderate intensity but haven't seen the changes in their body or fitness level that they're looking for. This phase helps you build strength and power so you can graduate to the more advanced exercises in Phase 5: Lean 15 Workout to get the lean, toned body you want.

Phase 1: Resistance Training (weeks 1-4) - Alternate between press-up supersets and kickback supersets, using dumbbells instead of barbells.

Phase 2: Strength Training (weeks 5-8) - Alternate between super squat supersets and single-arm dumbbell row supersets, using barbells instead of dumbbells.

Phase 3: Advanced Resistance Training (weeks 9-12) - Alternate between cable pulldown supersets and super squat supersets, using a variety of weight plates attached to one end of the cable.

Phase 4: Strength and Power (weeks 13-16) - Alternate between walking lunges and squat thrusts.

Phase 5: Lean 15 Workout (weeks 17-20) - Alternate between mountain climbers and glute bridges.

Phase 6: Core Challenge Workout (weeks 21-24) - Alternate between Russian twists and crunches with a medicine ball.

Chapter 8: The 15-Day Body of Your Dreams in Just 15 Minutes a Day (or Less)

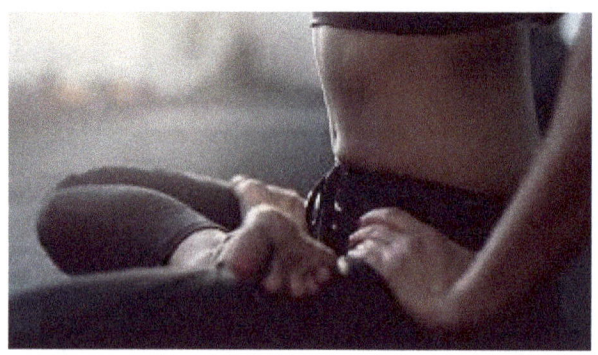

Part I. Introduction to the 15 Day Lean Body Program

The 15 Day Lean Body Program is a variation on the program designed by Martin Rooney and featured in his books. It is ideally suited for those who have a busy schedule but want to stay fit. The 15 Day Lean Body Program uses high intensity interval training (HIIT) to help you build lean muscle mass and burn fat faster than traditional cardio workouts. This quick workout can be done from anywhere with no equipment needed.

The 15 Day Lean Body Program relies on ideal bodyweight exercises to help you build lean muscle mass and burn fat in minimal time. The routines are inspired by the method used by the Australian Army Training Command to train soldiers for fitness and strength, with a specific focus on explosive strength. This method is used by elite athletes around the world.

To get you started, here is a sample routine from the 15 Day Lean Body Program. You can easily follow along with this program in your own home. Feel free to adjust reps or sets, if needed for your fitness level or schedule. Rest as needed between sets and feel free to repeat this workout as many times as you like within a 2-week period. If you need to break up the workout into smaller time periods to accommodate your schedule, that's fine.

• Workout 1 (15 minutes): one set each of squats, lunges, push-ups, and pull-ups

The Bodyweight Cardio Challenge Workout lists the bodyweight cardio exercises that you should use for this 2-week challenge. You will not do burpees because they are a high intensity exercise and therefore you cannot perform them on a day where you will also do bodyweight cardio. Be sure to choose one of the following exercises each time you do bodyweight cardio for the next 14 days.

Workout 2 (15 minutes): Burpee Challenge plus one set of push-ups

The Bodyweight Cardio Challenge Workout lists the bodyweight cardio exercises that you should use for this 2-week challenge. You will not do burpees because they are a high intensity exercise and therefore you cannot perform them on a day where you will also do

bodyweight cardio. Be sure to choose one of the following exercises each time you do bodyweight cardio for the next 14 days.

Workout 3 (15 minutes): two sets of each exercise

The Bodyweight Cardio Challenge Workout lists the bodyweight cardio exercises that you should use for this 2-week challenge. You will not do burpees because they are a high intensity exercise and therefore you cannot perform them on a day where you will also do bodyweight cardio. Be sure to choose one of the following exercises each time you do bodyweight cardio for the next 14 days.

Workout 4 (15 minutes): Bear Challenge plus push-ups

The Bodyweight Cardio Challenge Workout lists the bodyweight cardio exercises that you should use for this 2-week challenge. You will not do burpees because they are a high intensity exercise and therefore you cannot perform them on a day where you will also do bodyweight cardio. Be sure to choose one of the following exercises each time you do bodyweight cardio for the next 14 days.

Workout 5 (15 minutes): Mountain Climber Challenge plus pull-ups

The Bodyweight Cardio Challenge Workout lists the bodyweight cardio exercises that you should use for this 2-week challenge. You will not do burpees because they are a high intensity exercise and therefore you cannot perform them on a day where you will also do

bodyweight cardio. Be sure to choose one of the following exercises each time you do bodyweight cardio for the next 14 days.

Part II. The Fast Track to the Core Program

The Fast Track to the Core Program uses high intensity interval training (HIIT) to help you build lean muscle mass and burn fat faster than traditional cardio workouts. This 2-week program can be done from anywhere with no equipment needed.

The Fast Track to the Core Programs relies on ideal bodyweight exercises to help you build lean muscle mass and burn fat in minimal time. The routines are inspired by the method used by the Australian Army Training Command to train soldiers for fitness and strength, with a specific focus on explosive strength. This method is used by elite athletes around the world.

To get you started, here is a sample routine from the Fast Track to the Core Program. You can easily follow along with this program in your own home. Feel free to adjust reps or sets, if needed for your fitness level or schedule. Rest as needed between sets and feel free to repeat this workout as many times as you like within a 2-week period. If you need to break up the workout into smaller time periods to accommodate your schedule, that's fine.

- Workout 1 (15 minutes): one set each of squats, lunges, push-ups, and pull-ups

The Bodyweight Cardio Challenge Workout lists the bodyweight cardio exercises that you should use for this 2-week challenge. You will not do burpees because they are a high intensity exercise and therefore you cannot perform them on a day where you will also do bodyweight cardio. Be sure to choose one of the following exercises each time you do bodyweight cardio for the next 14 days.

Workout 2 (15 minutes): Burpee Challenge plus one set of push-ups

The Bodyweight Cardio Challenge Workout lists the bodyweight cardio exercises that you should use for this 2-week challenge. You will not do burpees because they are a high intensity exercise and therefore you cannot perform them on a day where you will also do bodyweight cardio. Be sure to choose one of the following exercises each time you do bodyweight cardio for the next 14 days.

Workout 3 (15 minutes): one set of each exercise

The Bodyweight Cardio Challenge Workout lists the bodyweight cardio exercises that you should use for this 2-week challenge. You will not do burpees because they are a high intensity exercise and therefore you cannot perform them on a day where you will also do

bodyweight cardio. Be sure to choose one of the following exercises each time you do bodyweight cardio for the next 14 days.

Workout 4 (15 minutes): Bear Challenge plus push-ups

The Bodyweight Cardio Challenge Workout lists the bodyweight cardio exercises that you should use for this 2-week challenge. You will not do burpees because they are a high intensity exercise and therefore you cannot perform them on a day where you will also do bodyweight cardio. Be sure to choose one of the following exercises each time you do bodyweight cardio for the next 14 days.

Workout 5 (15 minutes): Mountain Climber Challenge plus pull-ups

The Bodyweight Cardio Challenge Workout lists the bodyweight cardio exercises that you should use for this 2-week challenge. You will not do burpees because they are a high intensity exercise and therefore you cannot perform them on a day where you will also do bodyweight cardio. Be sure to choose one of the following exercises each time you do bodyweight cardio for the next 14 days.

Part III. The Fast Track to the Fat Burn Program

The Fast Track to the Fat Burn Program uses high intensity interval training (HIIT) to help you build lean muscle mass and burn fat faster than traditional cardio workouts. This 2-week program can be done from anywhere with no equipment needed."

The Fast Track to the Fat Burn Program relies on ideal bodyweight exercises to help you build lean muscle mass and burn fat in minimal time. The routines are inspired by the method used by the Australian Army Training Command to train soldiers for fitness and strength, with a specific focus on explosive strength. This method is used by elite athletes around the world.

To get you started, here is a sample routine from the Fast Track to the Fat Burn Program. You can easily follow along with this program in your own home. Feel free to adjust reps or sets, if needed for your fitness level or schedule. Rest as needed between sets and feel free to repeat this workout as many times as you like within a 2-week period. If you need to break up the workout into smaller time periods to accommodate your schedule, that's fine.

- Workout 1 (15 minutes): one set each of squats, lunges, push-ups, and pull-ups

The Bodyweight Cardio Challenge Workout lists the bodyweight cardio exercises that you should use for this 2-week challenge. You will not do burpees because they are a high intensity exercise and therefore you cannot perform them on a day where you will also do

bodyweight cardio. Be sure to choose one of the following exercises each time you do bodyweight cardio for the next 14 days.

Workout 2 (15 minutes): Burpee Challenge plus one set of push-ups

The Bodyweight Cardio Challenge Workout lists the bodyweight cardio exercises that you should use for this 2-week challenge. You will not do burpees because they are a high intensity exercise and therefore you cannot perform them on a day where you will also do bodyweight cardio. Be sure to choose one of the following exercises each time you do bodyweight cardio for the next 14 days.

Workout 3 (15 minutes): one set of each exercise

The Bodyweight Cardio Challenge Workout lists the bodyweight cardio exercises that you should use for this 2-week challenge. You will not do burpees because they are a high intensity exercise and therefore you cannot perform them on a day where you will also do bodyweight cardio. Be sure to choose one of the following exercises each time you do bodyweight cardio for the next 14 days.

Part IV. Wrapping Up with Fat-Burning Tips from Our All-Star Team

The Fat Burning Plan contains four fat burning workouts to help you create lean muscle mass and burn fat in minimal time. The routines in the program are inspired by the method used by the

Australian Army Training Command to train soldiers for fitness and strength, with a specific focus on explosive strength. This method is used by elite athletes around the world.

To get you started, here is a sample routine from the Fat Burning Plan. You can easily follow along with this program in your own home. Feel free to adjust reps or sets, if needed for your fitness level or schedule. Rest as needed between sets and feel free to repeat this workout as many times as you like within a 2-week period. If you need to break up the workout into smaller time periods to accommodate your schedule, that's fine.

- Workout 1 (15 minutes): one set each of squats, lunges, push-ups, and pull-ups

The Bodyweight Cardio Challenge Workout lists the bodyweight cardio exercises that you should use for this 2-week challenge. You will not do burpees because they are a high intensity exercise and therefore you cannot perform them on a day where you will also do bodyweight cardio. Be sure to choose one of the following exercises each time you do bodyweight cardio for the next 14 days.

Workout 2 (15 minutes): Burpee Challenge plus one set of push-ups

The Bodyweight Cardio Challenge Workout lists the bodyweight cardio exercises that you should use for this 2-week challenge. You will not do burpees because they are a high intensity exercise and therefore you cannot perform them on a day where you will also do bodyweight cardio. Be sure to choose one of the following exercises each time you do bodyweight cardio for the next 14 days.

Workout 3 (15 minutes): Bear Challenge plus push-ups

The Bodyweight Cardio Challenge Workout lists the bodyweight cardio exercises that you should use for this 2-week challenge. You will not do burpees because they are a high intensity exercise and therefore you cannot perform them on a day where you will also do bodyweight cardio. Be sure to choose one of the following exercises each time you do bodyweight cardio for the next 14 days.

Workout 4 (15 minutes): Mountain Climber Challenge plus pull-ups

The Bodyweight Cardio Challenge Workout lists the bodyweight cardio exercises that you should use for this 2-week challenge. You will not do burpees because they are a high intensity exercise and therefore you cannot perform them on a day where you will also do bodyweight cardio. Be sure to choose one of the following exercises each time you do bodyweight cardio for the next 14 days.

Chapter 9: Benefits Of 15 Minutes Workout

- One cannot complain that one does not have time to work out, in the busy schedule of life. 15 minutes robust workout technique is commonly being practiced by the working professionals to maintain their work life balance.

- The interval workout with high intensity is said to show better results as compared to normal cardio workout outs which stretch for longer duration.

- The person can decide the kind of work out one wants to plan, to suit his daily needs and his body characteristics.

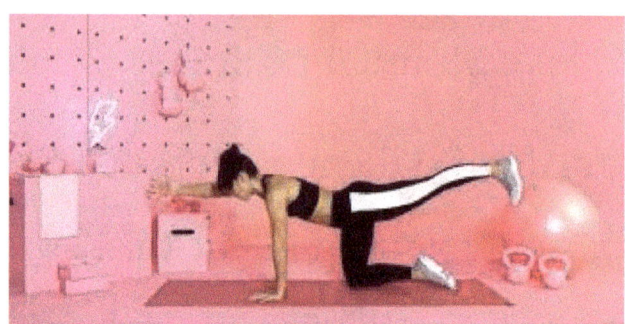

There Are Various Tips Which Needs To Be Followed Before Exercising

1. Start Slow

Any new thing has to be started with lower expectations as it takes time to get used to doing something new and also takes time to get results out of the same. For a start, one should do very basic exercises like running for 10 minutes on a daily basis for next three weeks. Body will need to get used to physical pressure and exercise. If someone starts with a heavy work out then he can seriously damage his internal organs because of excessive heat and sudden increase in body temperature.

2.   Change The Cycle

The exercise should be a onetime permanent set. The exercise should keep changing so that it does not get boring and monotonous. According to the purpose of the exercise one should also change the type and duration of exercise. For example if someone wants to increase the body muscle then he should limit his cardio exercise to a bare minimum and if someone is working out to get lean then his whole workout session should be dedicated to cardio exercises. In cardio exercises also one should take care of alternating the exercise on a daily basis. The person exercising in home can change the options from cycling to rowing to running on a treadmill, for 15 minutes.

3.   Separate Cardio From Strength Training

There are various strength building exercises and many cardio exercises which affects separately to the body. The cardio exercises affect the fat of the body and the strength gaining exercises are specific to body parts. If the person wants to gain strength in his hand or legs then he accordingly does crunches and squats to increasing the leg strength. Now running and cycling also is leg exercise but comes under cardio exercise. It is important to separate the two exercises and do not perform cardio exercise and leg strength increasing exercise in one day. This will lead to fatigue and the purpose of the exercise will not be solved.

4. Removal Of Fat Burning Zone Myth

Initially it was a common believe that a person need to exercise in 70-80 percent of his maximum heart rate to start the metabolism process and start losing fat. It was also a common believe that one will have to keep working out, in the above mentioned rate, for at least 20 minutes before the fat burning process starts. This, however, has been proven as a myth and now it is accepted that if a person follows interval workout sessions then he can definitely reduce his fat. The interval workout says that the workout should be done on various sessions of 15 minutes. This 15 minute session should be very intense and then after the session a person should take some rest. The metabolism process starts in those 15 minutes.

5. Practice Low Impact Exercise

There are a few exercises like running on asphalt floor or skipping. These exercises leave a lot of impact on the muscles of the body specially the feet muscles. These exercises lead to muscle breakage and it tears down the stamina to work out more. It is advisable to do intensive exercise but a low impact one. The exercises of this nature are cycling, swimming and running on elliptical machines.

6. 15 Minutes Interval Workouts

To reduce fat early one should to cling to interval workouts. These are the short and heavy sessions of workouts. In a shorter span of time one can lose more as compared to the regular cardio workouts. If a person does 20-30 minutes of interval workout, 2-3 times in a week then he reduces more as compares to 30-60 minutes of daily cardio workouts. The best part of interval workouts is that one keeps losing the body fat even after the workout session is not in the progress. The fat metabolism process is alleviated and it keeps happening for 48 hours after the work out session.

7. Change The Pattern And Time

Our body gets used to a workout. If a person is doing a particular kind of exercise at one particular time, on each and every single day, then the exercise will stop showing results after sometime. Let us take an example to understand it better. If a person is doing 3 sets of 10 squats each at 8am in morning, on a daily basis then after a month or so the body will get used to the pressure of 10 squats at 8am and thus will stop showing any results. That is why it is advised that a person should keep changing the number of sets he is doing, change the time of exercise and also the kind of exercise, from time to time. The change will give better results.

8. Body Toning In Interval Exercise

After the 15 minutes exercise session, all the stubborn fat is reduces and the skin is not visible as a loose skin. The interval workouts help in development of muscle in place of fats. This is the reason that, even after burning lot of fat the skin becomes tight as it has been transformed into muscles.

9. Exercise In Cool Area

It is commonly known and accepted that a person cannot exercise a lot in high degree temperature an. It is advised that the exercise should be done in cooler areas. If at all a person has to work out in high degree then he can cool his temperature around his neck and can work out for more time even in high degree. Wear an ice strap around neck region or wear a wet handkerchief around a neck region and run in treadmill. The duration will definitely increase vis s vis non cooling exercise.

10. Wear Comfortable Clothes

During work out wear something which does not absorb heat from outside and store in the body. for example if someone wear black color clothes during workout then this color cloth will absorb all the radiation from sun and will not reflect back. This will increase the heat within the body. The body is anyways heated up because of heavy workout and then if it socks more heat from outside then it will be dangerous for body. One should always take care of clothes and wear loose and light color clothes.

Conclusion

You now have the tools to workout without worrying about travelling or having access to a gym. You can workout anywhere at anytime. All you need is your bodyweight and determination. With these workouts, you can take your fitness to the next level by learning how to get fit, lean muscle mass and burn fat faster than traditional cardio workouts with minimal time.

You will be amazed at what your body is capable of doing when you challenge yourself with new workouts for fat burning. These workouts will help you burn maximum calories and get lean muscle mass too! If you would like to learn more about the secrets of fat burning then go here my website Bodyweight Cardio Training. You will learn more about fat burning workouts without needing to spend hours on the treadmill or run on a track. You can get fit without having to spend hours a day. You will learn the secrets of bodyweight cardio training to get lean muscle mass and burn fat in minimal time. So why wait. It's time to start your bodyweight cardio challenge now. Goodbye boring workouts for fat burning! Hello bodyweight cardio training for lean muscle mass and fat burning.

7-Minute Workout for Seniors

Simple Home Exercises to Reclaim Strength, Balance and Energy Above the Age of 60 (No-Equipment Needed)

Anphora Cooper

Table of Contents

Introduction 227

Chapter 1: The Benefits of Doing the 7-Minute Workout 229

   The 7-minute workout is beneficial in many ways 229

   Benefits of doing the 7 minute workout to the old: 230

   The 7-Minute Workout for Seniors has many benefits: 231

   The three strength training exercises are: 233

Chapter 2: How to do the 7-minute Workout 236

Chapter 3: Three Powerful Techniques to Make Exercise a Habit 242

   Technique 1: Habit Stacking 245

      What it is: 245

      How will this help me? 245

   Technique 2: Conditioned Cues 245

   Technique 3: Intrinsic Reward Statements 246

      What is it: 247

      How will it help me: 247

   Key takeaways 248

Chapter 4: Great Results at Home with Little or No Equipment 249

   Functional Training 249

   Exercising at Home 250

   Combination Approach 251

Chapter 5: The 7 Minute Workout for Seniors: Rest and Recovery 256

Early Recovery phase 256

The Late Recovery phase 257

Active Recovery, ... 258

Chapter 6: Tips for Family Members and Caregivers 261

Enthusiasm 262

Empathy 262

Encourage 263

Ease 264

Key Takeaways 267

Action Steps 267

Chapter 7: The Workout Routine 269

Here's a sample stretching, strengthening, and cardio routine 270

Chapter 8: Is There an Ideal Diet? 276

Popular Diets 277

The components of the Mediterranean diet: 279

Food Sources: Good and Bad 280

Chapter 9: Motivation and Commitment 284

The Motivation 284

The Commitment 285

Positive Reinforcements 286

Inspirational Quotes 288

Chapter 10: Questions and Answers 291

How to Improve Your Performance: 292

Questions and answers on the 7-minute workout for the seniors: 293

Conclusion 299

Introduction

7-Minute Workout for Seniors is a fitness book that specifically focuses on the benefits of exercise for seniors. The idea of this book is to provide information and inspiration to ensure that seniors can continue to live active, healthy lifestyles in old age. This book provides both a workout regime as well as advice on how to prepare for it. Because this book focuses on older individuals, it also includes some useful information about growing old, reminding readers that aging need not mean the end of physical activity and comfort with one's body.

This book has been written with the intention that it can be used by anyone, regardless of their educational background. It includes information on the importance of regular exercise for a healthy lifestyle and details of various exercises that can be carried out without any special equipment. These exercises are particularly geared towards individuals who may not have much strength or energy but with practice, can become more comfortable with their bodies and begin to move more independently. This book has been well-received by users because it does not require any sort of specific pre-existing condition in order to make use of its contents. It does not focus on fitness in terms of weight loss but rather, as a means to improve quality of life for older individuals. It has also been praised for its multiple useful tips which remind readers that the 7-minute workout is not just about getting fitter but also about being able to move more in general.

Chapter 1: The Benefits of Doing the 7-Minute Workout

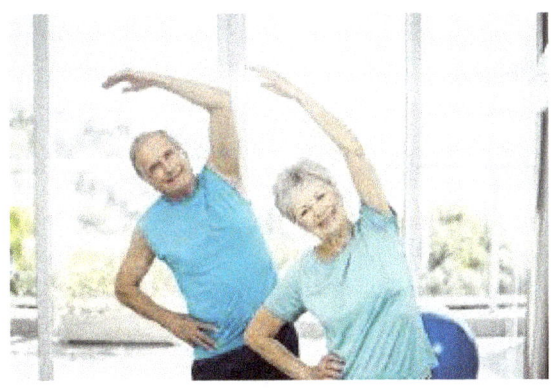

The 7-minute workout is beneficial in many ways.

The fact that the workout only takes seven minutes is great for working adults who do not have much time to work out but want to stay fit. This is also beneficial for children's after-school activities, as kids tend to be very busy and would not have the time nor patience to do a long workout. This is also beneficial because it requires only your body weight and no fancy equipment.

The 7-minute Workout could also be used to help individuals suffering from chronic diseases such as diabetes, hypertension, and heart disease by reducing their risk of developing certain diseases associated with sedentary lifestyles. It reduces the risk of developing other illnesses (e.g. obesity) that can lower your quality of life.

The 7-minute Workout is not just for adults; it is also beneficial to children and teens. It helps in fostering a healthy lifestyle early in life and ultimately lowering the risk of developing illnesses that are associated with sedentary lifestyles (e.g. heart disease, diabetes, obesity). Kids can do these exercises at home as often as possible because they only take seven minutes and they do not need expensive equipment.

The seven-minute workout is structured into four intervals. The workout has three different levels, each with their own workout routine.

I. Warm-up: Jumping jacks, High Knees, Butt Kicks and Star Jumps (each circuit for 30 seconds).

II. Strength Training: Squats (15 repetitions), Push-ups, Lunges (each circuit for 30 seconds). III. Core Strengthening: Crunches and Planks (each circuit for 30 seconds).

IV. Cool Down: Supermans and Back Extensions, Tricep Dips with a chair (each circuit for 30 seconds).

Benefits of doing the 7 minute workout to the old:

1) You will save yourself precious time in the mornings.

2) You will feel fresh and energized after your workout.

3) The workout is perfect for beginners.

4) It will help you build very lean muscle.

5) You can get very good results with this routine even if it is your first time working out.

6) It is a best way to maintain healthy weight.

7) It is an easy home workout, which requires just a pair of dumbbells, and a chin-up bar (or two chairs).

Gravity training utilizes the force of gravity as a resistance and does not require any special equipment or the purchase of expensive gym memberships.

Yoga is the practice of achieving physical, mental and spiritual balance through breathing, relaxation, and postures. Many people consider yoga as a way to reduce stress and improve overall health. Regular practice can be beneficial for flexibility, muscle strength, cardiovascular fitness, balance and coordination.

The 7-Minute Workout for Seniors has many benefits:

In order to improve performance in a physical activity it is necessary to do exercise. This does not mean that all exercise will increase performance in this activity it simply means it is necessary to do some exercise. Exercise can have many different benefits depending on the person's goals for their fitness program. In general exercise will strengthen our muscles and cardiovascular system which in turn will make us more fit. We often take for granted the many benefits we get from exercising. If you exercise regularly you will not only be healthier but happier as well. When we exercise our body releases endorphins which are said to make us feel good and happy. The endorphins also make us feel like having more energy too!

The 7-Minute Workout is said to be designed for seniors but can be beneficial to anyone who is a novice exerciser or has poor health, such as heart disease or diabetes. This workout consists of three rounds of seven exercises that should last about seven minutes in total. It is important to warm up before performing this workout and cool down after it as well. The author suggests that you should try to do this workout three times a week. The 7-Minute Workout for Seniors consists of 10 exercises. It takes only six minutes in total to do the circuit once. Perform one set of each exercise in the first minute and then one set of two exercises in the second minute, three sets of two exercises in the third minute and finally four complete rounds. These exercises are:

The core is a group of muscles that help stabilize your body during movement and keep it upright on both land and water. Strengthening your core muscles will help improve your performance in activities such as dancing, swimming, running or cycling. Core strengthening exercises usually target the lower back, upper back, abdominal muscles and hips.

The 7-Minute Workout for Seniors consists of three minutes of core exercises. The six exercises are:

The muscles in our body can be divided into two groups based on their location and function. Flexor muscles bend the joint and extensor muscles straighten it. There are some muscles that do both flexion and extension at the same time, such as the hip muscle. The 7-Minute Workout for Seniors consists of three minutes of strength exercises. These exercises target flexor and extensor muscles and help improve your performance in activities such as walking, running, swimming or golfing. The six exercises are:

The three strength training exercises are:

The last three minutes of this 7-minute workout is known as the cool-down and consists of three exercises. These exercises help relax your muscles after a hard workout :

These four sets together make up 6 minute circuit in a 7 minute workout. The book gives many reasons why we should exercise and participate in different physical activities such as dancing. The author states that one of the best ways to achieve a healthy body is by reducing our risk of developing many illnesses such as heart disease, obesity, diabetes, osteoporosis and depression. The author states that it is also important to eat a healthy diet because the food we eat can help our muscles recover faster after exercising or help them grow. The author also claims that by improving our health we can save money on medical bills and also have better quality of life.

The 7-Minute Workout for Seniors has proven to be beneficial throughout many stages of life, but particularly when beginning a fitness program or being diagnosed with heart disease or diabetes as stated in the introduction. This workout has also been proven to maintain muscle strength as we get older which is very important because it can improve balance and reduce the risk of falling which is one of the leading causes of death for seniors. This workout is also beneficial before and after a surgery. It can help with rehabilitation after the surgery and it will also help you get back into shape faster. This workout can improve cardiovascular fitness, balance, coordination, bone density and muscle strength. The 7-Minute Workout for Seniors is also beneficial for individuals who have chronic diseases such as diabetes, osteoporosis or heart disease because it can help reduce your risk of developing other diseases associated with sedentary lifestyles such as obesity or cardiovascular disease.

The 7-Minute Workout is designed to be done at home, but you can do this workout almost anywhere: at the gym, in your dorm room or in a hotel room. There are no special equipment needed to do this workout except for the following (if you don't have them at home) It is recommended that anyone who has just started exercising should begin by doing the exercises in the circuit three times and then working their way up to five times. It is also suggested that you progress from one circuit to another by increasing your repetitions (e.g., three sets of 10 each exercise). In order to improve your cardiovascular fitness you can do exercises such as jogging, walking, or cycling. Since you will be performing three circuits of this workout it is suggested that you perform the cardiovascular exercise for 10 minutes. The author suggests that for each circuit you should work up to about 80 percent of your maximum heart rate and then decrease it in order to recover. It is also suggested that the cool down should last about 1-2 minutes. It is also important that you drink plenty of water throughout each day and eat a healthy diet in order for your muscles to recover faster.

Chapter 2: How to do the 7-minute Workout

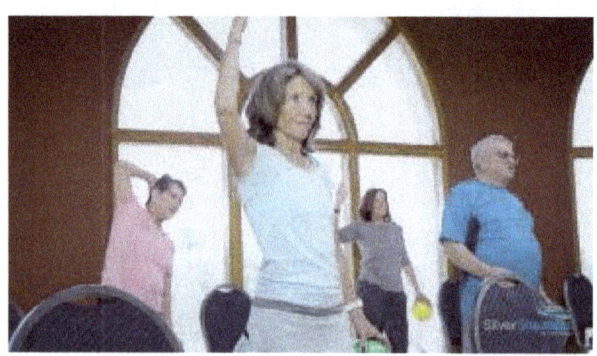

This introduces the reader to the different exercises that can be incorporated in the 7 Minute Workout. It describes a range of bodyweight exercises that can be carried out without any special equipment but with varying levels of intensity

For example:

1) Standard push-ups – performed on hands and toes on a hard surface such as a floor – can build strength, improve posture, and help prevent injuries. This is one of the most simple exercises that anyone can do anywhere at any time. This exercise can be made harder by performing a push-up on one's knees instead of the standard position.

2) Squats – performed in a standing position with the feet at hip distance apart and then bending down until the knee is at right angles or close to it. This will help to build strength in the core and lower body, as well as improving overall balance.

3) Lunges – performed in a standing position with one foot forward and one back. As you lunge, focus on keeping your upper body

straight and upright with your weight on the heel of your front foot. This will improve overall strength in the legs, improve balance, as well as working out different muscles depending on which leg is used during the lunge.

4) Planks – performed with the body in a straight line and supported on the hands and toes. This exercise is designed to strengthen the core and increase overall flexibility.

5) Crunches – this exercise can be done by lying on your back with your knees bent and feet flat on the ground, or alternatively, for those who are more mobile, it can be preformed by sitting up with legs crossed to build strength in the core.

6) Raises – this is another simple abdominal exercise that anyone can do anywhere at any time. It involves simply drawing one's shoulders up towards their ears, holding for a few seconds and then lowering back down again.

This also focuses on the importance of exercise to the aging population, who are often perceived as a sedentary population who are not as active. However, close examination reveals that there is an active senior population in old age and it is important to recognise this and continue the activity into old age. Despite this, activity levels do start to fall off after around 65 years of age, so it is important for seniors to continue exercising despite many thinking that they don't need the exercise in their older age. This chapter also explains the difference between physical activity and exercise, with exercise referring to any intentional movement done with a specific goal.

The difference between physical activity and exercise are:

1) Physical activity is any activity done outside of work that requires energy to perform

2) Exercise is a physical activity that has a specific goal. E.g. running to lose weight, swimming to improve stroke technique

3) Physical activity can be unpaid e.g. gardening, walking with friends, walking to work

4) Exercise is paid for e.g. gym, swimming lessons, aerobics class

It gives a thorough overview of the benefits of physical activity for seniors and focuses on the importance of being active as part of a healthy lifestyle, through both exercise and daily activities. By giving examples it tries to raise awareness in people about the necessity of staying active as part of an overall healthy lifestyle and that growing old does not mean having to stop doing things one enjoys or is good for them in general.

If you're 60 or older, the thought of becoming frail, suffering injuries from falls, and losing your independence is often a real worry, even if it isn't already happening. Our body changes as we age—and often in ways we don't like. We naturally lose 1-2 percent of our lean muscle mass every year after the age of 50. This gradual loss of muscle and strength is barely noticeable at first—until we wake up one day surprised that our physical ability is not what it used to be.

What if I could show you how to reverse muscle loss and reclaim your strength, balance, and energy faster than you ever thought possible?

It doesn't matter if you're 60 or 100 years old, or if you've been active or inactive your entire life. It doesn't matter if you're currently walking miles every day or struggling just to get up from a chair. It doesn't even matter if your health is perfect or imperfect. This book will show you how to transform your body and your life, no matter who you are, irrespective of your current state of health and fitness.

The book explains the core principle of the program: 'Use it or lose it'. It explains why this is fundamental to both staying healthy and preventing falls as you age. It presents the science behind how exercise can decline with old age and how exercise can prevent or at least minimise these declines. Furthermore, it gives examples of what exercises one can do as part of their program to combat these declines in physical abilities.

It discusses why balance is important for an active life and also goes through a number of ways one can improve their balance. It also has an entire chapter dedicated to the importance of staying physically fit in order to prevent falls. This chapter goes through what causes falls, common myths about preventing falls and the science behind why exercises can help you stay balanced. It also gives examples of exercises that can be used as part of your program and how often you should do them in order to stay balanced. During the last few years there has been an increasing body of research on the topic whether brain training programs designed to improve cognitive functions such as memory, attention and decision-making are effective and reliable. The term does not include persons administered anesthesia or other psychoactive drugs while they are in an operating room, recovery room, intensive care unit or any other environment related to the practice of surgery or medicine. The term neurocognitive aging is the same as normal age-related cognitive decline. The main difference is that normal age-related cognitive decline is more global and diffuse, whereas neurocognitive aging involves areas of the brain that are more or less impacted than others.

Neurocognitive decline does not include gradual change in personality over time which happens with normal aging called "normal personality reorganization". Consequently, neurocognitive decline can occur independent of personality changes. One distinctive aspect of neurocognitive aging is that it substantially interferes with the individual's ability to pursue meaningful and purposeful activities during middle and late adulthood. As a result, the process of aging often leads to considerable disability and dependency in individuals who are otherwise physically healthy.

Neurocognitive decline is not a disease. It is simply a natural process that everyone experiences as they age.

According to the research conducted by Eyal Shahar and colleagues on elderly individuals who regularly spent time outdoors, cognitive functioning was observed to be greater in those individuals compared to those who did not spend as much time outdoors. This was connected to activity of the hippocampus, which is an area of the brain associated with spatial knowledge, memory, and emotion. Other research has found that when elderly patients who suffered from Alzheimer's were exposed to nature for two months they showed visible improvements in brain functioning. This included increases in activity of the hippocampus, cerebellum, and superior parietal lobule, which are areas of the brain associated with memory. Staying physically active is important for everyone, but it's especially vital for older adults who are more at risk of falling and having other injuries. This book provides a series of 12 exercises that can be done in just 7 minutes and that will increase strength, improve balance, build coordination, and more. Each exercise takes only a few minutes to learn. Already in the first week of doing the program you will be able to see great results in your body, and over time you will transform your fitness level and your confidence level!

Chapter 3: Three Powerful Techniques to Make Exercise a Habit

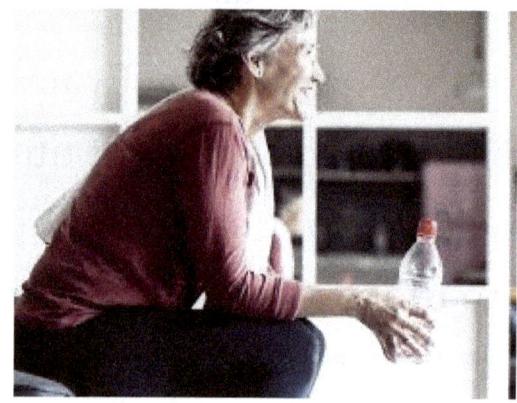

So you know from the previous 2 chapters that exercise is important and it will help you achieve your health, fitness and weight loss goals faster.

However, to make sure exercise becomes a habit, you need to use a specific approach. On this chapter I'll explain to you the 3 powerful techniques that will ensure your success. These techniques are: Decide what to exercise Focus on one thing at a time Implement the right rewards system

1. Decide What To Exercise This is so important! Don't just let yourself go or do what feels good at the moment. Instead, decide on the type of exercise program that you will do. For example, your goal is to lose weight, so instead of just running every day for 30 minutes, decide to do interval running. You may think interval training is just another way of exercising but it's not! If you want to gain more knowledge about interval training (and why I believe this type of training is the best) read Born To Run by Christopher McDougall. So "decide what to exercise" doesn't necessarily mean

you need to get a gym membership or equipment (although those things can help). Even if there's no gym nearby or you are too busy, all you really need are your body and your mind.

2. Focus On One Thing At A Time Decide what to exercise. You have to decide everything at once. So for example, if your goal is to lose weight and look better, decide that you will do the following: Interval running 3 times a week Weight training 3 times a week Yoga 1 time a week 15 minute meditation Daily water consumption of 2 liters Start with step 1! Don't worry about the others yet. It's important that you focus on only one thing at a time and when you've completed it, move on to the next one. So you may ask me: "How do I know which one to focus on first?" That's a great question. The answer is to ask yourself what's the most important for your situation. If you are overweight, it's very likely that exercise will help you burn more calories and thus lose more weight. So maybe put the interval running first and then move on to weight training later when you can fit it into your schedule. Decide what to exercise, this is half of the battle!

3. Implement The Right Rewards System The best thing about having a goal (like losing weight) is not just reaching it but also achieving smaller rewards along the way. This will keep you motivated and push you to stick to your plan. You can also use these rewards to make yourself feel better about yourself! Here is a list of rewards that I recommend: Decide on the 1st reward you will give yourself (could be a new pair of workout shoes or a nice

dinner) Make sure your rewards are limited (don't go overboard with them, choose something reasonable like two rewards for every 5 pounds) Find ways to enjoy these benefits, like eating a nice meal at the mall or window shopping

Now go out there and find a cool exercise program that's right for you. Make sure it's something you enjoy doing and can do regularly.

Technique 1: Habit Stacking

Habit stacking is a technique that will force you to do a series of habits. Our brain is lazy, which is good from one perspective, because once we've learned something it'll be easier for us to repeat it in the future. However, just like all other things, our brain needs some kind of stimulation so we stay on top of things. Habit stacking helps us with this by forcing us to initiate several habits at once and then take the actions needed to complete them.

One powerful application of habit stacking for exercise is a method called Run-Walk-Run .

What it is:

You alternate running with walking, so in other words you run and then walk. By doing this, you are able to exercise more efficiently and burn more calories.

How will this help me?

The answer to this question is really simple: if you walk more than you run, your heart rate and breathing will slow down instead of speeding up like when running. This means that your heart has to work less hard for the same amount of time. The result of this is that your body will burn fewer calories on a given period of time than if you were running all the time.

Technique 2: Conditioned Cues

This is an interesting technique that will allow you to prepare your mind for exercise and make it into a habit. It's very similar to how Pavlov's dog was conditioned to salivate in anticipation of food.

What is it?

You associate certain cues with exercising. For example, if you want to work out at the beach, then you may decide that when you start seeing the ocean, it's time for your run or walk workout. The idea is that once you start feeling that cue, your body (and your brain) will automatically prepare for exercise and you'll have a better chance of staying active throughout the day.

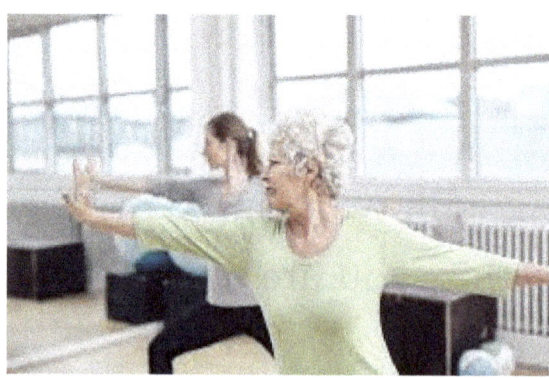

Technique 3: Intrinsic Reward Statements

This technique is somewhat similar to habit stacking but it's also a little bit different. The basic idea here is that you intersperse different activities into your workout. For example, instead of just running for 30 minutes, you can interleave jogging with jumping jacks. This will help you stay alert and active throughout the whole workout session.

Another example would be for weight training. Instead of just doing the same thing over and over again, you could do an exercise (like bench presses), then do something different (like bicep curls), then go back to bench presses and so on. This will keep your mind from getting bored and thus keep you more active throughout the workout session.

What is it:

This technique, pretty much like its name suggests, involves creating a visual representation of your exercise routine. This could be something like a poster with pictures to remind you of your workout plan for the week. Just seeing that reminder everyday can be enough to force you to act on it. Another option is to use an app or software program that helps you make the chart so you don't have to do the work yourself. There are two programs I really recommend: My Fitness Pal (fitnesspal.com) and Fitocracy (fitocracy.com).

How will it help me:

This technique is a bit different from the previous two. But personally I find it the most powerful of them all because you can use it no matter what your goal is. The idea behind this is that you create a goal and then you stick to it by posting it somewhere public where everybody can see. This way, if you don't start working towards your goal, people will notice and you'll feel bad about not taking action. Next time we'll be talking about how to make exercise a habit so stay tuned! In the meantime, keep on working out.

Key takeaways

Creating an exercise schedule that works best for you is not enough. That's why you need to learn how to make exercise a habit and start doing it without putting too much effort into it. I've outlined three techniques that will help you do just that:

1. Implementation Intentions

2. Habit Stacking

3. Visualization

There's one more technique you can use, which is a combination of the first two: First, make your schedule and then create an implementation intention to start implementing the schedule. This way you can make sure your schedule is not just sitting on a piece of paper but it's actually working for you.

Chapter 4: Great Results at Home with Little or No Equipment

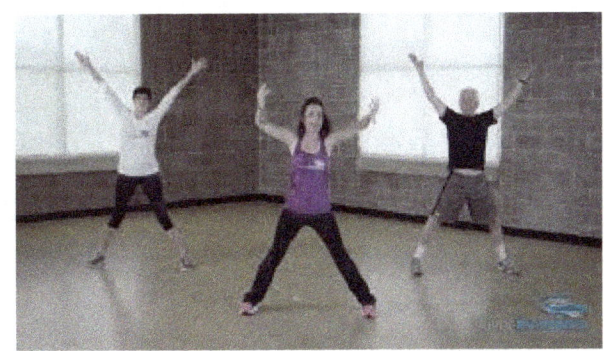

During the coronavirus pandemic, workout equipment flew off the shelves, with millions of people scrambling to put together a home gym because fitness centers were closing across the country. Equipment such as weights, exercise bikes, and rowers were out of stock for months. The good news is exercise can be just as effective without a gym or workout equipment. You can easily achieve the same results—or even better—exercising at home with little or no workout equipment using something called "functional training."

Functional Training

Functional training mimics activities or specific skills you perform at home, at work, or in sports to help you thrive in your daily life. This kind of training is effective because it uses different muscles simultaneously and also emphasizes core stability — the control of muscles around the abdomen and back that protect your spine when you move. For example, performing squats with a chair trains the same muscles you use when you rise from a chair, pick up an object from the ground, climb stairs, or hike up a mountain.

Many fitness and rehabilitation experts, including myself, have known for a while that functional training is the most effective way to train. Finally, the research is catching up with our observations. Functional training has now been shown in multiple studies to produce results that are superior to most other forms of exercise for diverse groups of people, including young military personnel, middle-aged females with low back pain, and (of course) older adults.14

One study demonstrated that high-intensity functional training was safe and effective for improving balance and independence in individuals aged 65 and older who had dementia and were living in nursing homes.15 Another showed that functional training significantly improved the golf swing and fitness level of golfers aged between 60 and 80 years old.16

By training your muscles to work functionally, you'll prepare your body to perform well in a variety of tasks that are important to your daily life—and you can do it at home with the aid of "equipment" readily available, such as a backpack filled with canned goods, to increase the difficulty level of exercise.

Exercising at Home

There are several additional benefits to exercising at home versus going to a gym:

- The ease and convenience of exercising at home removes demotivating barriers. You don't have to drive to the gym, change your clothes in a room full of strangers, or wait for workout equipment to free up.

- The gym can be an intimidating place for some older adults. But self-consciousness or fear of what others may think is not a concern with functional training at home.

- For older adults who don't function well enough to leave home without assistance, going to the gym can be difficult or impossible. Exercising at home is the only way for these people to improve strength, balance, and function.

- The price tag of a gym membership can be an obstacle for many older adults on fixed incomes. Cost is not an issue with workouts at home that require little or no equipment.

Combination Approach

The real secret to this program is the integration of higher-intensity training (discussed in the last chapter) and functional training, adapted for older adults. You won't find this combined approach to exercise for older adults in many other places, but it's a method that will allow you to safely and quickly achieve great results at home with little or no equipment.

You may be wondering at this stage why you couldn't just do something else that needs no equipment—such as walking—for exercise. It's certainly true that walking is another form of functional training that doesn't require equipment and can be good for your health, but in the next chapter I'll explain why walking alone isn't enough to reverse age-related muscle loss.

Key Takeaways

- You can easily achieve the same or even better results exercising at home with little or no workout equipment using "functional training."

- Multiple studies have shown functional training to produce results that are superior to most other forms of exercise for diverse groups of people, including older adults.

- The real secret to this program is the integration of higher-intensity training with functional training adapted for older adults. It will allow you to safely and quickly achieve great results at home with little or no equipment.

Action Steps

- Prepare yourself for exercising at home by making sure you have the following items handy:

    o A backpack filled with heavy items (such as canned goods) for resistance.

    o A pair of five-pound ankle weights.

- If you're a family member or a caregiver for an older adult you'd like to help with exercise, prepare them for exercising at home by making these items available.

- Only use a pair of five-pound ankle weights, and not heavier ones, when you exercise. Lighter weights are more comfortable and will allow you to perform the exercises with better form.

It is important to note that the risk of a heart attack or stroke is highest in the first three days following a sudden change in physical activity levels. Therefore, it is critical to speak with your doctor before starting an exercise program.

- It's best to begin with about 3 minutes of exercise per session and build up gradually over the next few weeks to as much as 10 minutes at a time.

- It's not necessary to do all twelve exercises every week—in fact, you may find that you feel more comfortable adding just two or three new exercises each week.

- Workout every day at home (ideally) or 3 days/week for optimal results from this program.

- It is important to incorporate a warm-up and a cool-down into your home workout to prevent injury and experience greater benefits.

- Perform each exercise with perfect form at least two or three times before moving on to the next exercise.

- Check with your doctor before starting this program.

- To maintain gains obtained from working out, it's vitally important to resist the urge to take breaks when you can easily fit in a workout routine.

What you need to know about training at home:

- It's common, especially in older adults, to experience some aches and pains after a workout. If this occurs, stick with the program, but cut back on the intensity of the exercise or change the duration of your workout until you can tolerate it well. For example, instead of doing 10 minutes of walking, do 5 minutes walking and 5 minutes of easy stretching.

- If you experience chest pain that is not relieved by medicine or does not go away within a few minutes after stopping exercise, it may be a sign of unstable angina (a warning sign for heart attack). Seek medical help right away.

- If you experience tightness, pain, or numbness in the area of your chest that does not subside within a few minutes, it may be a sign of a heart attack that is occurring right now. Seek medical help right away as this can cause sudden death.

- If you experience sudden dizziness or nausea while exercising and it does not go away within a few minutes after stopping exercise, it may be a sign of an inner ear disturbance—a warning sign for stroke. Seek medical help right away.

- If you have high blood pressure or a history of heart attack or stroke, consult with your doctor about starting this program slowly with lower-intensity exercise and shorter duration at first. I recommend that these individuals start by doing 3 minutes/day of exercise and progress gradually by adding 1 minute of exercise each week. When they can tolerate 10 minutes per day, they can return to the regular program.

- If you have osteoporosis, a history of broken bones, or if you have ever fainted due to low blood pressure, it is very important to talk to your doctor about having an exercise stress test before starting this program. Most individuals older than 60 who have had heart attacks or strokes should also have an exercise stress test.

- Seek a doctor's advice if you have had any of the following conditions and are considering starting this program: hypertension, heart condition (including an irregular heart beat), diabetes, chronic lung disease, joint problems, or smoking.

- If there is any doubt about your ability to exercise—due to health problems or medications you are taking—you should consult with your doctor before starting this program.

Chapter 5: The 7 Minute Workout for Seniors: Rest and Recovery

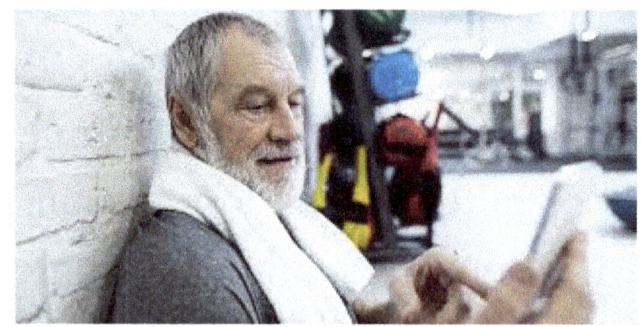

This chapter focuses on the rest and recovery aspect of the 7-Minute Workout. The author explains that using the seven minutes to work out is not enough and that a routine such as this must be complemented by adequate time spent in rest and recovery. The rest and recovery aspect of the 7-Minute Workout is made up of three phases: Early Recovery, Late Recovery and Active Recovery.

Early Recovery phase

In the Early Recovery phase, the author recommends that you should get off of the floor or out of the water and sit for a short period of time. Here you can even perform some gentle stretching if this is comfortable. If you exercise in a pool or at the beach, then you can simply stay in the water and float on your back for a few minutes. In this phase, it is recommended that you refrain from any intense exercises. It is said to be important to separate this from the Early Recovery phase and perform it about twenty minutes after the workout is completed.

While moving into the Late Recovery phase, it is recommended that you perform energizing exercises such as arm circles or leg swings. This should be done for approximately 2-3 minutes after the workout has ended. It is also recommended that you continue your rest and try not to sit or lay down for long periods of time. The author suggests that you may want to begin performing gentle stretching at this point but stay away from Yoga or Pilates because they increase flexibility which can cause an imbalance in your muscles and joints. The Late Recovery phase should last about five minutes.

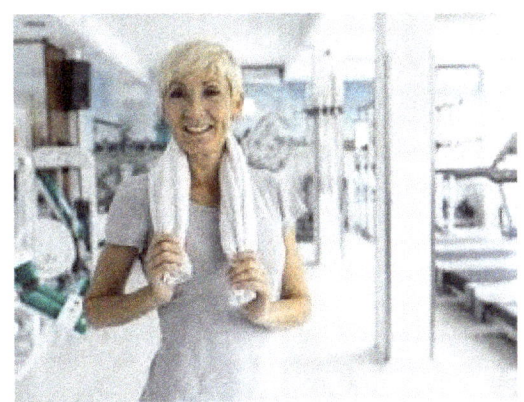

The Late Recovery phase

This is the most important phase of rest and recovery because this is when your body becomes ready for its next major stress or challenge. The author explains that we are not at a state where we need to be worrying about recovering our bodies in this case as we already have. It is said that during this time it can be important to get sufficient amounts of sleep because during sleep our body heals itself with increased blood flow. During sleep the blood flow to our brain increases by 50% and we achieve REM sleep in which our concentration levels are better and the brain consolidates memories.

Active Recovery,

This period of training is low intensity and consists mainly of aerobic activity such as walking or cycling to improve circulation around the body. The author explains that this should be done for 30-60 minutes. This helps return blood that has built up in our muscles after exercise back into the blood stream. If Active Recovery Phase is not followed, there is a danger of overtraining because after several days of hard training you will have fatigue which could lead to illness, injury or burnout.

When your muscles and joints are in the Early Recovery phase, you can try to strengthen your connective tissues with exercises such as yoga. By doing this the author says you can improve flexibility and prevent injury which could otherwise be caused by a weak or brittle muscle. The author states that performing yoga for a short 3 minutes after a Workout is enough to significantly increase circulation, heart rate and respiration which will enhance recovery in addition to reducing stress and anxiety.

The second half of this chapter provides many different methods of how you can improve rest and recovery such as stretching, self massage, tapping and meditation. The final section of this chapter is titled "Yoga, Strengthening and Balance." The author explains how the practice of yoga (see Yoga) has proven to be beneficial for all ages. The author then explains how yoga can be incorporated into a 20 or 30-minute workout because we are all short on time and this is the main reason why the 7-Minute Workout for Seniors was invented in the first place.

The author explains that a good warm up should last 10–20 minutes and can include exercises such as walking, jogging, cycling, swimming or any other activity that gets your heart rate up. After this the author says that we should do a circuit of exercises for 7 minutes. The 7-Minute Workout for Seniors consists of 10 exercises that should be performed in a circuit style. In the first minute perform 1 set of each exercise and then in the second minute perform 2 sets, and so on until you reach 7 sets. The author states that it is possible to perform this workout in both a fasted state or after eating. The author then provides a table with each exercise listed along with the page number where it can be found and details about how much weight to use/how deep to go and also which muscles that exercise works out. The circuit consists of the following exercises:

The last exercise in this circuit is a plank. The author states that the plank is a good way to measure progress because it has no weight requirement and only takes ten seconds to complete. The author says that when you begin the 7-Minute Workout for Seniors this plank should be held for 15–20 seconds and you should work towards increasing it to 60–90 seconds. This second half of this chapter contains information about Yoga, Strengthening and

Balance. The author explains how by practicing yoga you can strengthen your muscles, improve balance, relieve stress and have more energy at rest. The author also claims that practicing yoga will improve your flexibility. The chapter starts off with a description of Yoga. The author then explains how yoga can be incorporated into a 20 or 30-minute workout and how to do each movement correctly. The following yoga postures are described with pictures to help you see the correct form:

Next are all the exercises that you can use if you are not doing a yoga routine such as squats, lunges, push-ups, bridges, calf raises and planks. These exercises will help strengthen the muscles and increase bone density in your body. You can do this along with walking or any other aerobic activity because it is said that "muscle strengthening is key to improving muscular health. Strength training has been linked to delaying the onset of physical disabilities, which reduces the risk of falling and fracturing bones." The last section in this chapter is for Balance Exercises. The author then explains how "improving our balance can reduce our risk of falling, which is important as falls are one of the leading causes of injuries and death among older adults." By doing these exercises you will be able to get your muscles ready for challenging movements that you will perform if you take dance lessons or go hiking with friends.

Chapter 6: Tips for Family Members and Caregivers

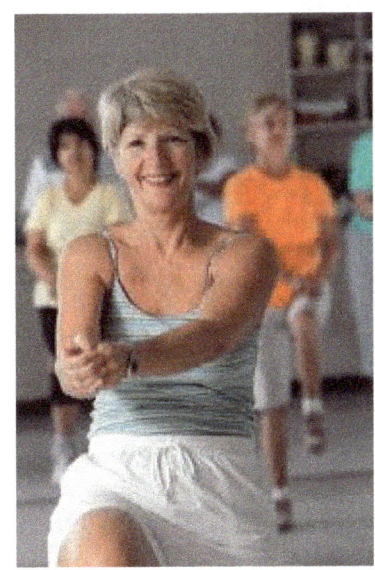

Older adults with memory issues or who lack the motivation to exercise will need help from another person.

Although we never want to force someone to exercise when they don't want to, persuasion is sometimes necessary because a persistent lack of movement leads to serious issues, such as debility, bed sores, and injuries from falls.

Older adults with memory issues or who lack motivation may have a difficult time starting and sticking with an exercise program. But I've found it becomes less challenging once exercise becomes routine, and changes in strength, balance, and energy become apparent after a few weeks.

The key to persuasion is a simple process I've created called the four Es: enthusiasm, empathy, encouragement, and ease. This process takes only a few minutes and has been effective with even my most exercise-resistant clients. Let's explore each step in detail.

Enthusiasm

Richard Simmons, the semi-retired American fitness instructor known for his eccentric and energetic personality, is a great example of enthusiasm at its best. It's difficult not to feel pumped up and motivated to move when you watch him.

So the first step in motivating someone is to be enthusiastic. Your enthusiasm is contagious, and it can shift another person's energy level and desire to exercise in powerful ways. To make enthusiasm work, you have to authentically feel it and express it in your words and body language.

Try to authentically feel and express enthusiasm in your voice, posture, gesture, and facial expression while saying something like, "Dad, it's time to exercise. It'll only take six minutes, and you'll feel great afterward. Let's do it!" If you encounter any resistance, move to the next step.

Empathy

The second step is to feel and express empathy: the ability to understand and share the feelings of another. It's important because a person is more likely to be open to your suggestions when they know you've understood and considered their perspective.

So to feel empathetic, you should know the common reasons why an older adult may not want to exercise: They may have lost hope that things will ever get better. They may be fearful that the aches and pains they experience daily will get worse if they exercise. They may feel constantly exhausted and don't know if they have the energy needed to exercise.

Whatever the reason, start by stepping into their shoes and feel what they may be feeling. Then express your understanding through your words and body language. Try to authentically feel and express empathy in your voice, posture, gesture, and facial expression while saying something like, "Dad, I can understand that you're feeling exhausted, and the aches that come with your age don't help. I also wonder if you've lost some hope that things can get better." It helps to pause for several seconds at this point to tune in to feelings that may be coming up for you and the other person. Then, move to the next step, which is to encourage the person.

Encourage

After feeling and expressing empathy, it's time to encourage the person to exercise.

For this to be effective, I suggest doing two things. First, understand the person's personal values and bring them into this step. A person's values can be things like determination or hope or respecting authority figures such as doctors. Second, remind the person of the benefits of exercise that are important to them. These benefits can be things like feeling more energized after exercising, gaining the ability to live more independently, feeling happier because they can avoid hospitalizations, or having more energy playing with the grandchildren.

Whatever the reason for exercising, keep it positive, and express it with passion in your words and body language.

Use this step to authentically feel and express passion in your voice, posture, gesture, and facial expression while saying something like, "Dad, you always told us growing up that sometimes things will get worse before they get better, and having hope will get you through these times. It's no different getting your body working better through exercise. Remember how much you want to get back to gardening? What do you say?" If the person still isn't convinced to exercise at this point, it's time for the final step.

Ease

The fourth and final step is to ease into exercise. Use this when the previous steps haven't persuaded the person to take action. Your goal is to make exercise something the person can try for a few repetitions to see how it feels, knowing they can stop any time.

To make this step work, I recommend you first openly acknowledge that the person really doesn't want to exercise. Then suggest that they try just a few repetitions of one exercise to see how it feels. Tell them they can stop any time.

Perform this step with enthusiasm, and encourage the person to continue exercising after they've started. With enthusiastic encouragement, most people won't stop exercising once they've begun and may even surprise you with their new motivation.

Use this step to authentically feel and express enthusiasm in your voice, posture, gesture, and facial expression while saying something like, "I totally understand that the idea of exercise doesn't sit well with you right now, but let's just do five chair squats and see how it feels. I'll help you, and you can stop any time if you don't want to continue after that. Come on, let's start now."

As the person approaches the fifth repetition of the exercise, enthusiastically encourage them to continue by saying something like, "Wow, you're looking really strong! I'm amazed by how well you're doing! Keep going, I know you've got it in you!"

Applying the four Es takes only a few minutes and has been effective with even my most exercise-resistant clients. However, at times, nothing you do will persuade someone to exercise. It's best to yield to the person's wishes in these moments.

Fortunately, just two or three good workout sessions a week is enough to see improvements with this program in most adults. That may be all you will get out of someone who really doesn't like to exercise—but after a few weeks, they may be more motivated after noticing improvements in their strength, balance, and energy. So stay positive and be patient.

Key Takeaways

- The four Es can help persuade the person to exercise: enthusiasm, empathy, encouragement, and ease.

- The first step is to be enthusiastic. Your enthusiasm is contagious, and it can increase another person's desire to exercise. To make enthusiasm work, you have to authentically feel it and express it in your words and body language.

- The second step is to feel and express empathy: the ability to understand and share the feelings of another. A person is more likely to be open to your suggestions when they know you've understood and considered their perspective.

- The third step is to encourage. Understand the person's values and include them in your conversation, and remind them of the benefits of exercise that are important to them.

- The fourth and final step is to ease into exercise. Use this strategy when the previous steps haven't persuaded the person to exercise. The goal is to make exercise something the person can try for a few repetitions to see how it feels, knowing they can stop any time.

Action Steps

- If you're a family member or a caregiver for an older adult you'd like to help with exercise, practice the four Es a few times on your own to get comfortable with the method before using it to persuade them to exercise

Chapter 7: The Workout Routine

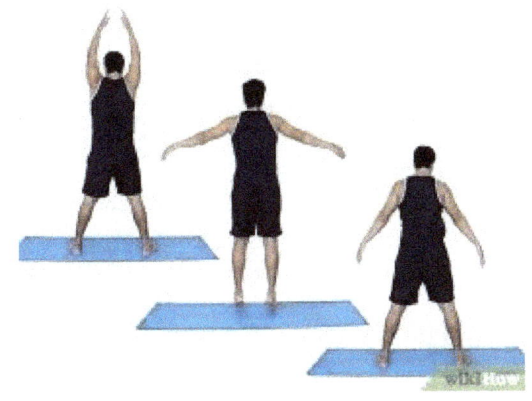

In this section, the exercise moves laid out in the previous chapter will be put together for a routine that will be suited to your fitness level. Determine your fitness level and take the fitness test in Chapter 4. Doctors recommend having at least 150 minutes of physical activity a week. Spread out over the week, that's 30 minutes of activity for five days. Workouts are great but you'll have to give your body time to adjust and recover. Two days of rest and recovery can be inserted midweek or during weekends. From 150 minutes, you'll build up to 225 minutes, and eventually 300 or more minutes a week. These routines aren't set in stone. As you progress and learn, and get used to the exertion, you'll have the confidence and the personal knowledge to mix and match exercise moves you feel would best suit your body's strength and endurance levels.

The plan is to do each level consistently for four weeks until you've increased your stamina and endurance, and could do more reps, more sets for longer periods. Before starting on any fitness routine, make sure that you've assessed your health and fitness functionality with the tests in Chapter 4. If you fall within the below average range, you'll start at the beginner level with a focus on 70% cardio to improve your stamina and 30% strength training. If you've an intermediate level result, the ratio is 60% cardio and 40% strength training. For those with results in the expert level, it'll be equal parts cardio and strength training. The routines outlined here are also adaptable to where you're most comfortable doing your exercises. A fifth of the exercises could be done outdoors - walking, cycling, and swimming. The rest can be done at home or at the gym. The exercise equipment needed is also minimal or easily adaptable with items readily found at home.

Work needs to be done to develop mobility and stamina if your fitness test shows below average results. Perform 15 minutes of stretching exercises to improve mobility and 15 minutes of simple cardio workouts.

Here's a sample stretching, strengthening, and cardio routine.

3 minutes of warm-up stretches

- Perform 2 times, Upper Back Stretch
- Perform 2 times, Chest Stretch
- Perform once on either side of the neck, Neck Stretch
- Perform 2 times, Sit and Reach Stretch
- Perform once for each leg, Inner Thigh Stretch

- Do 1 set of 16 reps, Shoulder Circles
- Do 1 set Hand Stretches

8 minutes of muscle strengthening & balance exercise

DAY 1

- 2 sets of 10 reps for each leg, Side Leg Raise
- 2 sets of 16 reps, Seated Shin Strengtheners
- 2 sets of 8 reps, Pliés
- 2 sets of 10 to 15 reps, Front Arm Raise
- 2 sets of 5 reps for each side, Side Bends
- 2 sets of 8 reps, Tummy Twists
- 2 sets of 10 reps for each leg, Knee Extensions
- 2 sets of 10 reps for each hand, Wrist Curls
- 4 sets of 15-20 steps, Toe the Line
- 2 sets of 10-second Flamingo Stands for each leg
- Perform 3 Clock Reaches for each side

DAY 2

- 2 sets of 10-second Flamingo Stands for each leg
- 2 sets of 10 reps, Side Leg Raise

- 2 sets of 10 to 15 reps, Front Arm Raises
- 2 sets of 5 reps for each side, Side Bends
- 2 sets of 8 reps, Tummy Twists
- 2 sets of 10 reps for each hand, Wrist Curls
- 2 sets of 10 to 12 reps, Bicep Curls
- 2 sets of 16 reps, Seated Shin Strengtheners
- 2 sets of 8 reps, Pliés
- 2 sets of 10 to 15 reps, Wall Push-Ups
- 2 sets of 10 reps for each leg, Knee Extensions

DAY 3

- 2 sets of 5 reps for each leg, Leg Lifts
- 2 sets of 15 reps, Seated Knee Lifts
- 2 sets of 10 reps, Knee Extensions
- 2 sets of 10 to 15 reps, Front Arm Raises
- 2 sets of 10 reps for each hand, Wrist Curls
- 2 sets of 10 to 12 reps, Bicep Curls
- 2 sets of 16-second Single Limb Stance with Arm for each leg
- Perform 3 Clock Reaches for each side
- 2 sets of 8 to 10 reps, Modified Burpees

- 2 sets of 5 reps for each side, Side Bends
- 2 sets of 15 reps, Seated Twists

DAY 4

- 2 sets of 5 reps for each leg, Leg Lifts
- Perform Bicycles for 30 seconds, rest, then go another 30 seconds
- 4 sets of 15-20 steps, Toe the Line
- Do 2 turns on the Speed & Agility Drill ladder
- 2 sets of 10 reps for each hand, Wrist Curls
- 1 set of 10 reps, Dumbbell Upright Row
- 2 sets of 10 to 15 reps, Wall Push-Ups
- Perform 3 Clock Reaches for each side
- 2 sets of 8 to 10 reps, Modified Burpees
- 2 sets of 8 reps, Pliés
- 2 sets of 16 reps, Seated Shin Strengtheners

DAY 5

- 2 sets of 10-second Flamingo Stands for each leg
- 2 sets of 16-second for each leg, Single Limb Stance with Arm
- 2 sets of 16 reps, Seated Shin Strengtheners

- 2 sets of 10 reps for each leg, Side Leg Raises
- 2 sets of 8 reps, Pliés
- 2 sets of 5 reps for each side, Side Bends
- 2 sets of 8 reps, Tummy Twists
- 2 sets of 15 reps, Seated Twists
- 1 set of 10 reps, Dumbbell Upright Row
- 2 sets of 10 to 15 reps, Wall Push-Ups
- 2 sets of 8 to 10 reps, Modified Burpees

15 minutes of cardio exercises

- 5 minutes marching in place
- 10 minutes of brisk walking

ALTERNATE CARDIO A

- a 15-minute bike ride or

ALTERNATE CARDIO B

- 5 minutes easy resistance on a stationary or elliptical bike
- 10 minutes medium resistance on a stationary or elliptical bike

2 minutes of cool down stretches

- Perform 2 times, Upper Back Stretch
- Perform 2 times, Chest Stretch

- Perform the cool down routine below:

1. March in place for 30 seconds.
2. Step your right foot forward to a lunge position and rest your hands on the middle part of your right thigh. Lunge forward taking caren't to let your knee go over your toes.
3. You should feel a bit of a stretch on your left calf. Hold the position for 16 counts. Switch positions and repeat step number 2 with your left leg.
4. Step your right foot behind and rest your hands on your hands on your right knee. Slowly bend from the waist pushing your buttocks backward and up.
5. You should feel a bit of a stretch on the back of your left thigh muscles. Hold the position for 16 counts. Switch positions and repeat step number 4 with your left leg.
6. March in place for 60 seconds. Stand with a wide stance and spread your arms upwards to stretch. Sweep your arms down to the side and raise them up again. Repeat this move for 8 counts.

Chapter 8: Is There an Ideal Diet?

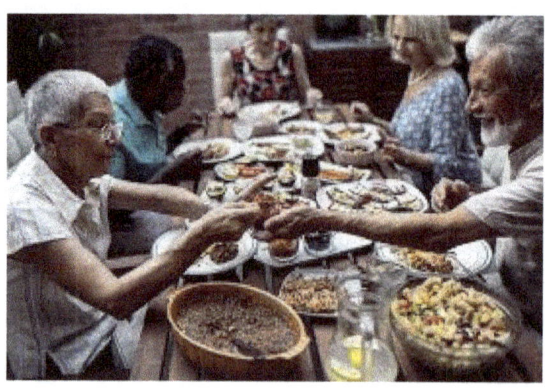

Walk into a bookstore and look for the section for books on diet. You will need time just to read the titles because the number of diets that are recommended is extensive. There are several reasons for this:

➤ Many people need help and guidance on weight loss and for managing conditions and illnesses: diabetes, heart disease, hypertension, cancers, immune disorders, and psychological problems among others.

➤ There is generally a belief that there is a magic diet, a silver bullet solution to lose weight, build muscle, cure disease, and live longer.

➤ Diet is all about eating, and people generally take eating very seriously as evidenced by the size of the cookbook section at the bookstore.

Let's take a quick look at some of the diets that are popular today, but with the understanding that while there are responsible ways to help with weight control and prevent or alleviate certain diseases, there is no single amazing diet that is the solution for everyone's problems. There is no "one size fits all" die because each of us has our own unique physiology, our own metabolic rate, our own sensitivities.

Popular Diets

Fasting has emerged recently as a way to health, happiness and a longer life, but you need to know that while the research involving worms and mice has been encouraging, the studies involving humans are mostly in the early stages. The more common approaches are intermittent fasting, conducted on a daily, repeating basis, such as the 16:8 fasting diet, which allows eating during an eight-hour period (e.g., 8 a.m. to 4 p.m.), and nothing to eat for the next 16 hours (4 p.m. to 8 a.m.). There are stricter versions, like 18:6. Alternatively, some try prolonged fasting, going for 24- or even 48-hour fasts, followed by a day of unlimited eating. People who practice this tend not to overeat on the non-fast days because their stomachs shrink a bit during the fast period,

➢ As a weightlifter seeking to build muscles, fasting diets are not advised for you.

Paleo diets harken back to paleolithic, simpler times when our distant ancestors were hunter-gatherers and ate "off the land," which means whatever they could find. This inspires diets today that avoid all refined and processed foods (which is commendable)

and based on foods that our bodies evolved over millions of years to digest effectively.

A paleo diet limits foods like dairy products, grains and legumes, and potatoes that became available when farming and agriculture started around 10,000 years ago. Added salt is also avoided. Overall, the paleo diet is acknowledged as healthy and wholesome as long as the ratios of macronutrients are respected, and a diversity of foods is included so that adequate amounts of vitamins and minerals are included.

Keto diet, short for ketogenic, has a very specific objective: rapid weight loss through stimulation of fat burning. This is achieved by following a very high-fat, very low- carbohydrate diet, essentially replacing the carbs with fats. This results in a metabolic condition called ketosis, which is highly efficient in using stored and dietary fat, instead of carbs and stored glycogen, for energy. You burn fat; you lose weight. Another quality is the conversion of fat stored in the liver to ketones, which supply energy to the brain. Also, the keto diet has been shown to lower blood sugar and insulin levels, which may contribute to the prevention or reduction of diabetes and other disorders. Other benefits are a feeling of fullness (satiety) that reduces cravings to eat or snack and improved mood. Studies of the longer-term effects of keto and other very low-carb diets are underway.

While the keto diet appears to be effective for weight loss, it may not include sufficient protein for building muscle mass; at least 30 percent of your diet should be protein.

Mediterranean diet. Let's conclude with a diet that is not only gaining broad acceptance, but it is the closest to the ideal diet everyone is searching for. It includes a wide range of wholesome and great-tasting foods, is affordable, is credited by the medical community as being heart-healthy, and may help slow the onset of many other diseases, from diabetes to cancer.

This diet is based on the practices of long-term residents of the Mediterranean Basin, including parts of Italy, Spain, and France, who tend to live healthier, longer lives. But importantly, these people practice a lifestyle that includes not only diet, but also being physically active all their lives, keeping their weight at normal levels, and having a positive attitude towards life.

The components of the Mediterranean diet:

- A variety of fresh vegetables, fresh and dried fruits, nuts, and seeds, whole grains and cereals, fish, lean meat in small servings (e.g., six ounces), moderate quantities of dairy (mostly as cheese), eggs, extra virgin olive oil, and wine, mostly red, consumed in moderation.

Whatever diet you choose, remember that as a weightlifter and builder of strength and muscle, you need sufficient protein in your diet, and you should select foods that are low in saturated fats. Avoid salty, processed foods, fried foods, and anything containing large amounts of sugar. The next section details the good and bad sources of foods.

Food Sources: Good and Bad

The types and sources of the three macronutrients have been discussed in detail, but to summarize, here is a quick checklist of the good and the bad. While this chapter has been devoted to helping you to understand the foods that are most beneficial to your health and to improve your level of physical fitness, build muscle and make you stronger, there are sources of carbohydrates, proteins, and fat that you should avoid. To help your dietary planning, we've listed both the recommended sources of your macronutrients and the foods that have been designated as undesirable and potentially harmful.

According to nutritionists at MD Anderson Cancer Center:

Recommended carbohydrates sources include:

➢ Dairy products, including milk, yogurt, and cottage cheese, but with a preference for low-fat or non-fat since full-fat dairy products are high in saturated fats and calories. Non-dairy substitutes made from soy, almonds, and oats are also good sources of carbs. Dairy products also provide high-quality complete protein.

➢ Vegetables, which can be eaten without limitation since they are low in calories and rich in vitamins and minerals. Select a variety of colors (green, yellow, red, purple) which will provide a diversity of micronutrients.

➢ Fruits are high in natural sugars (which is why they taste sweet) and micronutrients. Fruit should be eaten without added sugar and in natural, solid form to preserve pulp, which adds valuable fiber. Many juices have added sugar and the pulp has been removed.

➢ Beans, peas, and lentils, known as legumes, provide high levels of carbohydrates, plus fiber and many of the 20 amino acids that comprise protein.

➢ Whole grains, including whole wheat, rye, buckwheat, spelt, corn, and oats, are high in carbs and are excellent sources of vitamin B and fiber. Refined grains do not have these added qualities.

Carbohydrate sources to avoid:

➢ Refined flours and sugar, found in crackers, most breads, cookies, breakfast cereals, and sugar, in most fruit juices, soft drinks, most athletic performance beverages, and candy.

Recommended protein sources include:

- Beans, including black, pinto, and kidney beans, plus lentils and soy products. Except for soy, the proteins are incomplete and need supplementation with grains and cereals.

- Nuts and seeds, including nut butters (sugar-free versions).

- Whole grains, including quinoa, rye, wheat, spelt, corn, and soy, with the caveat that the amino acids do not comprise complete protein.

- Animal protein from meat, poultry, fish and seafood, dairy, and eggs.

Protein sources to avoid:

- Processed meats, like sausages, salami, bacon, frankfurters (hot dogs), and canned lunch meats.

- Consumption of lean red meats should be limited to 18 ounces per week.

Recommended fat sources include:

- Vegetable oils, especially extra virgin olive oil, avocado oil, and canola oil, and secondarily, oils from corn, sunflower, and safflower.

- Fatty fish, notably coldwater salmon, tuna, mackerel, and sardines.

- Flax seeds, chia seeds, avocados, and olives.

➢ Nuts and seeds, and again, natural nut butters, no sugar added.

Fat sources to avoid:

➢ Fried foods, which are made with refined flour and absorb large amounts of oils that contain trans fats.

➢ Animal sources, including full-fat dairy like milk, butter, yogurt, cream cheese, and the fats on meats and poultry.

➢ Vegetable oils from coconut and palm sources, shortening (used in baking), soft tub margarines, and most packaged baked goods (read the labels for fat content).

Now, on to Chapter 7 and dismissing some common misconceptions about working out, getting into shape, building muscles, and gaining strength when you are 60-plus.

Chapter 9: Motivation and Commitment

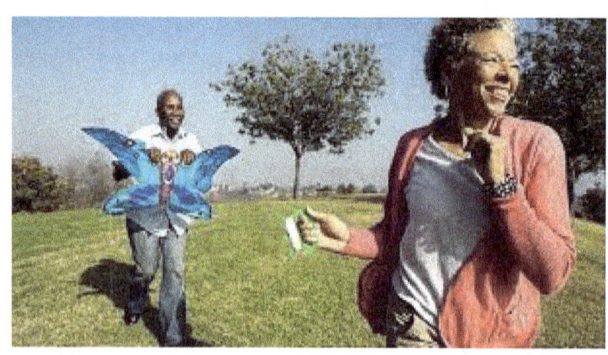

An important part of your long-term muscle and strength-building program is mental. Of course, it will be the weights, the reps, the sets, and the rests in between that will give you the lean muscle mass you want, but your state of mind will determine if you actually get started and if you will go the distance for the months and years of exercise it will take. Rome wasn't built in a day, and your impressive physique won't happen immediately.

The Motivation

In the initial chapter and at other points in this book, the importance of motivation was established as an incentive to getting your weightlifting and fitness program underway. No one can make you get into a regular, well-planned weightlifting program; you have to have the resolve and enthusiasm to take charge of your body, your health, and your appearance:

➢ If you have read this far, chances are good that you get it, "you're in."

➢ You imagine yourself lifting the barbells and dumbbells, doing the push-ups and pull-ups, the planks, the squats, and the splits.

➢ You feel committed to cardiovascular conditioning to help melt the extra pounds while you invest in your health and longevity.

➢ You feel better looking in the mirror in anticipation of the bigger, defined muscles you are going to build.

The Commitment

But will you have the determination and discipline to go the distance, to continue regularly with your bodybuilding and strengthening practices? Motivation is important at the beginning, but you need to have the discipline to stick to the routine even on days when you just don't have the drive, when you say, "I'll do it tomorrow."

You need to transcend the forces that hold you back, to break free of the constraints, and be committed no matter how tired or uninspired you are at that moment. Only then can you keep on track to meet your fitness and strengthening goals.

Commitment to succeed as a weightlifter, who builds muscle, who loses fat and excess weight, starts in the mind, which is the most effective and persuasive tool that will help you achieve your bodybuilding objectives. A positive attitude and the determination to work through the toughest movements will carry you through the worst of it with grit. Those who fail to make it, who give up, who quit, may be tough physically but don't have the mental toughness. Remember that your body will follow your mind.

Successful weightlifters at every level of training have developed positive thoughts to get themselves to the gym, to pick up the first weight of the session, to get through it with a full effort, no matter how tired or busy they were. You can adopt these thoughts, make them yours, let them carry you to the workout, and through the work, every time.

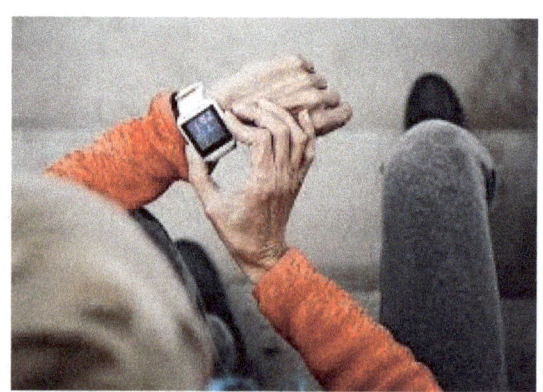

Positive Reinforcements

1. I'll just do a half-workout today, take it easy.

This works when you're tired and helps to get you started. In almost every case, once you get started and warmed up, you get into the movements, do all the reps, and go all the way. It's a little psychological game that you can play on yourself, and somehow it continues to work time after time. As it has been said, "just showing up is 90 percent of success," so just get those workout shoes and shorts on, get to a machine or a weight, and start out slowly. You'll warm up and keep going.

2. The solo mountain climber's focus and discipline.

When you are heading up the side of Yosemite's El Capitan, climbing without ropes or tools, there is no looking up or down, no thinking about what's coming or how hard it will be. The same applies to weightlifting when the only thing that matters is what you need to do at that moment: focus on the now. Another advantage of being in the moment while working out is the clearing of your mind, in a meditative way, so that all distractions are ignored. You will be calmer, and by paying close attention, your form and posture will be better, and you will be less likely to cause an injury.

3. The mirror, the scale, and the tape measure.

The numbers don't lie, exaggerate, or try to please your ego. They are the reality that will testify to the depth and duration of your commitment to building your body, getting your weight where it belongs, and getting that gut flatter. Start with a benchmark set of measurements, and check in every week. Look at yourself in the mirror without criticism or disappointment and just take notice of how your pecs (chest muscles) and abdominals look: a little soft, a layer of fat. Same for the arms and legs. Weigh yourself before breakfast, and write down the number each week, or daily if you prefer. Same for the tape measurement. Over time, you will see and record progress, and that will help solidify your commitment to your long-term objectives.

Inspirational Quotes

1. "Tough times don't last, but tough people do." — **Richard Shuller (2020).**

This quote applies to all aspects of life but has found special appreciation among professional lifters who push to their absolute limits. But especially for you as you are beginning weightlifting and conditioning, there are times when it isn't fun, like that last pull-up or barbell curl. Your thighs may be burning after three sets of squats or splits, and that last set of dumbbell rows may have you breathing pretty hard. But every time the set is over, and the rest begins, the pain and burning feeling subsides, and the workout always ends with a feeling of work well done, a sense of satisfaction. You are tough and getting tougher.

2. "To be a champion, you must act like a champion." — **Lou Ferrigno (2020).**

Lou Ferrigno, a champion weightlifter who played the Incredible Hulk, contributed to this recommended mindset because he believes that strength comes from within. A championship attitude is attainable by all of us if we believe in ourselves and envision the well-muscled, well-defined body we are working to achieve. But it goes further: If you want to become a well-built bodybuilder, you need to work out like one. Positive thinking is essential to motivate and inspire you, but without hard work and the determination to give it your all, positive thinking is just a dream.

3. "Don't wish it were easier. Wish you were better." — **Jim Rohn (2020).**

The thought leads us to expect that the workout, the lifting and pulling, the squatting and dipping, needs to be intensive, to challenge us. That leads to the realization that if it's easy, it's not being done right. You need to work to challenge your muscles to the point that muscle cells and fibers are damaged and need to self-repair through hypertrophy. The attitude that will carry you from passive to proactive is the recognition that it's a simple formula: strength is directly proportional to the effort that is invested in each workout. Of course, a hard workout can be followed in two days by a less intensive workout to aid recovery, but then be sure to make the next workout more intensive. It will pay off in the long-term.

4. "It never gets easier. You just get stronger." — **Unknown (2020).**

The idea is to add weights progressively when you can handle more without reducing reps, sets, or rest intervals. For example, head over to the dumbbell rack, and pick up a heavy weight you can do just one rep of a bicep curl or at most two. Do you wish you could do more reps? Find the weight you can lift or curl for eight reps and have the patience and confidence to know that in a reasonable time, with discipline, you will advance gradually from the lighter weight to the heavier ones and beyond. Just follow the basic practice of lifting weights that max out at eight to 10 reps, do the three sets, and be sure to rest between sets and between workouts.

5. "You have to be at your strongest when you're feeling at your weakest." — **Unknown (2020).**

This inspiration encourages weightlifters and cardio athletes to reach deep inside for the strength that they know is there. Imagine that you are a runner who is training for a marathon or other long-distance competition. The only time you can train is early in the morning before work, even in the cold and dark of winter. You need to roll out of bed at 5:30 a.m., wash your face, put on your running shoes, head outside, hit the road, and run into a biting cold headwind. What does it feel like to go through this, day after day, for months? This is what inner strength is all about, and it illustrates, in the extreme, what someone chooses to do to reach an objective. You probably will not have to work out under such an extreme condition. You'll be indoors, warm, lifting weights you can manage, and working to a reasonable, yet difficult peak of effort. But think of that runner in the dark, cold, early morning, and let it carry you to a better effort each day.

Chapter 10: Questions and Answers

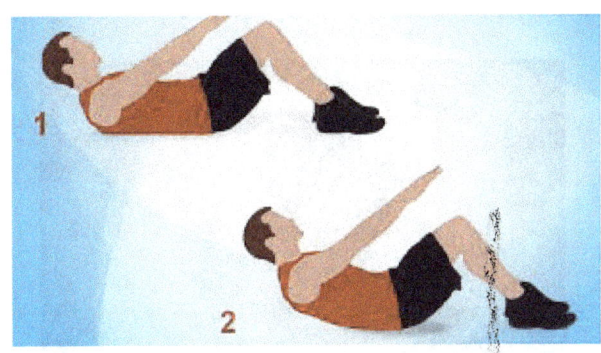

In order to stay fit the authors of the 7-Minute Workout suggest that you do this workout three times a week. The best time for you to do this workout is probably before or after breakfast, lunch or dinner. Even though you will only be performing circuits 2 and 3, it is suggested by the author that you consider doing circuit 1 too in order to warm up gradually.

The 7-Minute Workout for Seniors is a very beneficial workout routine for anyone. It is especially beneficial for people who are just beginning to exercise or individuals who have been diagnosed with heart disease, diabetes or osteoporosis. It is beneficial for people who are just beginning to exercise because it will help them become more fit and healthy. It is beneficial for people who have been diagnosed with heart disease, diabetes or osteoporosis because it can help reduce their risk of developing other diseases associated with sedentary lifestyles such as obesity or cardiovascular disease. This workout can also be used to improve muscle strength, balance and coordination. The 7-Minute Workout for Seniors is a great workout routine for individuals who are just beginning a fitness program or persons who want a simple and easy workout routine that helps them stay fit.

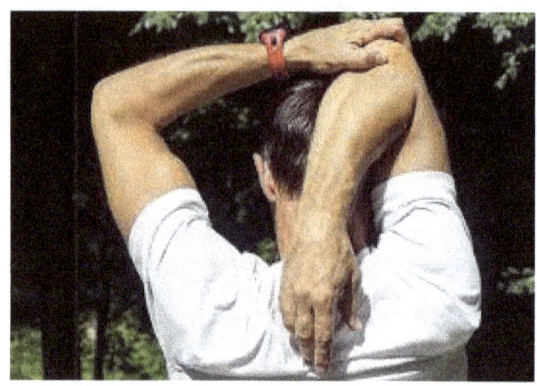

How to Improve Your Performance:

1) Always remember that you should warm up before doing any exercises.

2) The 7-Minute Workout for Seniors consists of four sets of exercises. For each set do 3 minutes (or 5 minutes in case you are doing circuit 2) with no rest in between the exercises.

3) The warm up should last about five minutes. It is recommended that you pick exercises that make your muscles feel a slight burning sensation and that also help you warm up slowly.

4) The 6 exercises consist of 1 minute, 2 minutes, 3 minutes and 4 minutes respectively. In order to learn more about how to do these exercises it is suggested by the author to check out the book titled "The 7-Minute Workout."

5) The cool down consists of three exercises and should last about two minutes.

6) You should drink plenty of water every day. At least one liter will be sufficient for the average person.

7) Eat a healthy diet to ensure adequate supplies of protein, carbohydrates and fats for your muscles. Also, eat plenty of different fruits and vegetables to ensure that you will get all the vitamins and minerals you need.

8) Plan to work out at different times in your week so you won't become bored or irritated by this workout routine. The book also suggests that you find a friend with similar goals as you do to help motivate yourself to include a fitness routine in your life regularly.

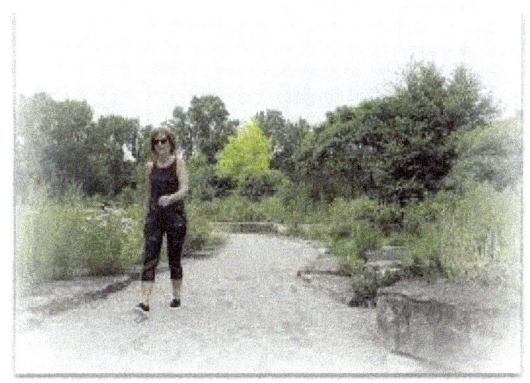

Questions and answers on the 7-minute workout for the seniors:

1. Can men do this workout?

This workout is be particularly beneficial for men. By doing this workout regularly the author of the book claims that it can help prevent heart disease and diabetes as well. This routine has also been proven to maintain muscle strength as we get older which is very important because it can improve balance and reduce the risk of falling which is one of the leading causes of death for seniors.

2. What are some other benefits of doing this workout?

This particular routine is good because it helps you improve your balance, coordination and bone density. It also helps you strengthen your cardiovascular fitness, muscles balance, coordination, bone density and muscle strength.

3. How many sets of exercises do I need to do?

The book suggests that you should do three sets of each exercise for about a minute. You also should perform each circuit three times before progressing to the next one. Progressing from one circuit to another by increasing your repetitions (e.g., three sets of 10 each exercise). The warm up should last about five minutes and you should work up to about 80 percent of your maximum heart rate and then decrease it in order to recover. It is also suggested that the cool down should last about 1-2 minutes. It is also important that you drink plenty of water throughout each day and eat a healthy diet in order for your muscles to recover faster.

4. Does the 7-Minute Workout for Seniors put a lot of pressure on my joints?

This workout routine is designed to be gentle for your joints because it is low impact and no knee or ankle weights are required.

5. How much space do I need to do this workout?

Since the 7-Minute Workout for Seniors consists of only three exercises that can be done at home or in other small places, it will not take up much space at all! It is very easy to do this workout routine.

6. What is the difference between circuit 1 and 2?

Circuit 1 consists of exercises that target your muscles and help them recover after performing other exercises. Circuit 2 consists of strength training exercises that target flexor and extensor muscles in order to improve your performance in activities such as walking, running, swimming or golfing.

7. Will I get bored doing this workout routine?

It is recommended by the author to use different times in your week for working out so you won't become bored. You may also want to find a friend with similar goals as you do to help motivate yourself.

The 7-Minute Workout for Seniors is a very beneficial workout routine for anyone. It is especially beneficial for people who are just beginning to exercise or individuals who have been diagnosed with heart disease, diabetes or osteoporosis. It is beneficial for people who are just beginning to exercise because it will help them become more fit and healthy. It is beneficial for people who have been diagnosed with heart disease, diabetes or osteoporosis because it can help reduce their risk of developing other diseases associated with sedentary lifestyles such as obesity or cardiovascular disease. This workout can also be used to improve muscle strength, balance and coordination. The 7-Minute Workout for Seniors is a great workout routine for individuals who are just beginning a fitness program or persons who want a simple and easy workout routine that helps them stay fit.

- This book will benefit you because it will help you improve your health by reducing your risk of developing many illnesses. The seven exercises contained in this book will help relax the muscles after a hard workout and also improve your cardiovascular fitness, balance, coordination, bone density and muscle strength.

- This workout is very beneficial because it does not take up much space at all! This routine consists of three sets of 6 exercises in order to be completed within seven minutes. It is very easy to do this workout routine. It can be done at home, the gym or even in a hotel room.

- This workout routine will help you improve your cardiovascular fitness because it contains exercises that target your muscles and help them recover after performing other exercises. Also, this routine helps relax the muscles after a hard workout and also improves your cardiovascular fitness, balance, coordination, bone density and muscle strength.

- This workout routine will help you stay fit because it can help prevent heart disease and diabetes. It can also develop your muscles strength as well.

- This routine helps improve muscle strength, balance and coordination. This workout also has been proven to maintain muscle strength as we get older which is very important because it can improve balance and reduce the risk of falling which is one of the leading causes of death for seniors.

- The 7-Minute Workout for Seniors consists of four sets of exercises that are all targeted for different parts of the body such as the chest, back, shoulders, arms, hips and thighs or legs. The warm up consists of three exercises in order to be completed within five minutes. The 6 exercises of this routine consist of 3 minutes, 4 minutes, 1 minute and 2 minutes respectively. In order to learn more about how to do these exercises it is suggested by the author to check out the book titled "The 7-Minute Workout."

- The cool down consists of three exercises and should last about two minutes.

- This workout routine has also been proven to maintain muscle strength as we get older which is very important because it can improve balance and reduce the risk of falling which is one of the leading causes of death for seniors.

- Information about why you should drink plenty of water everyday in order for your muscles to recover faster.

- Eat a healthy diet that provides you with adequate supplies of protein, carbohydrates and fats. Also eat plenty of different fruits and vegetables to ensure that you will get all the vitamins and minerals you need.

- Mix up your workout routine. Make sure that you plan to work out at different times in your week so you'll never get bored or irritated by this workout routine.

- You should drink plenty of water every day and eat a healthy diet in order for your muscles to recover faster.

Conclusion

This workout routine will improve your health by reducing your risk of developing many illnesses such as cardiovascular disease, osteoporosis and diabetes. This workout will help relax the muscles after a hard workout and also improve your cardiovascular fitness, balance, coordination, bone density and muscle strength. This program is very beneficial because it does not take up much space at all! It can be done at home, the gym or even in a hotel room.

This workout routine will help you improve your cardiovascular fitness because it contains exercises that target your muscles and help them recover after performing other exercises. Also, this routine helps relax the muscles after a hard workout and also improves your cardiovascular fitness, balance, coordination, bone density and muscle strength.

This workout routine will help you stay fit because it can help prevent heart disease and diabetes. It can also develop your muscles strength as well. This routine helps improve muscle strength, balance and coordination. This workout also has been proven to maintain muscle strength as we get older which is very important because it can improve balance and reduce the risk of falling which is one of the leading causes of death for seniors. The 7-Minute Workout for Seniors consists of four sets of exercises that are all targeted for different parts of the body such as the chest, back, shoulders, arms, hips and thighs or legs. The warm up consists of three exercises in order to be completed within five minutes. The 6 exercises of this routine consist of 3 minutes, 4 minutes, 1 minute and 2 minutes respectively. In order to learn more about how to do these exercises it is suggested by the author to check out the book titled "The 7-Minute Workout."

This cool down consists of three exercises and should last about two minutes.

This workout routine has also been proven to maintain muscle strength as we get older which is very important because it can improve balance and reduce the risk of falling which is one of the leading causes of death for seniors.

This workout routine has also been proven to maintain muscle strength as we get older which is very important because it can improve balance and reduce the risk of falling which is one of the leading causes of death for seniors.

This workout can help prevent heart disease and diabetes as well. It can also develop your muscles strength as well.

This workout routine will help strengthen your cardiovascular fitness, balance, coordination, bone density and muscle strength. Also, this routine helps relax the muscles after a hard workout and also improves your cardiovascular fitness, balance, coordination, bone density and muscle strength. This workout routine will help you stay fit because it can help prevent heart disease and diabetes. It can also develop your muscles strength as well.

The 7-Minute Workout for Seniors is a very beneficial workout routine for anyone. It is especially beneficial for people who are just beginning to exercise or individuals who have been diagnosed with heart disease, diabetes or osteoporosis. This exercise program is very beneficial because it does not take up much space at all! The exercises that are contained in this book will help improve your health by reducing your risk of developing many illnesses such as cardiovascular disease, osteoporosis and diabetes.